Welcome

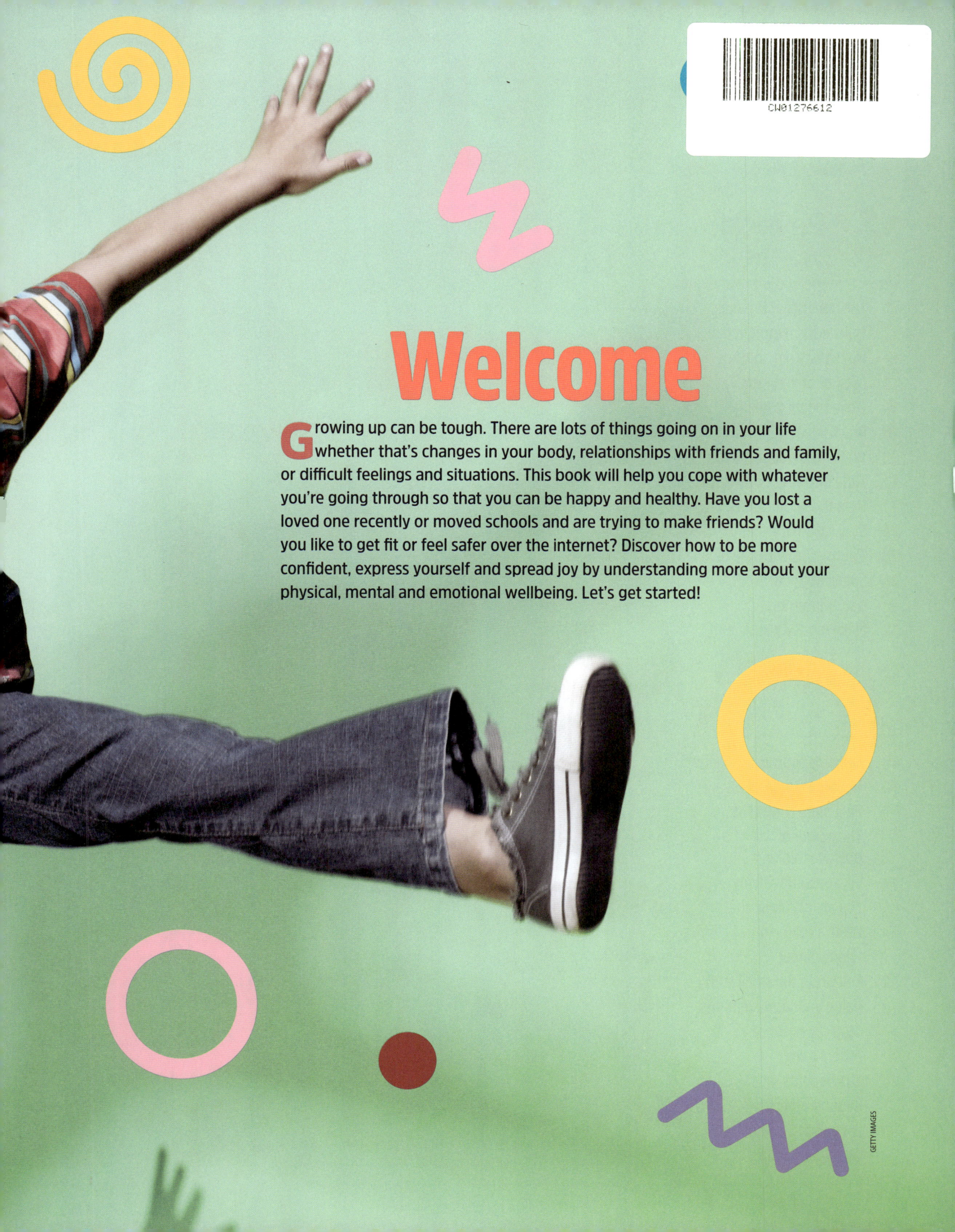

Growing up can be tough. There are lots of things going on in your life whether that's changes in your body, relationships with friends and family, or difficult feelings and situations. This book will help you cope with whatever you're going through so that you can be happy and healthy. Have you lost a loved one recently or moved schools and are trying to make friends? Would you like to get fit or feel safer over the internet? Discover how to be more confident, express yourself and spread joy by understanding more about your physical, mental and emotional wellbeing. Let's get started!

CONTENTS

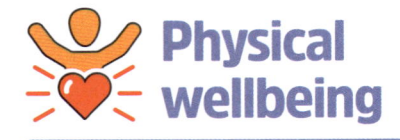

Physical wellbeing

10	The benefits of breakfast
12	Make easy overnight oats
13	Make tasty egg muffins
14	Look after your gut
16	Move to feel good
18	Practise yoga
20	Walking is a superpower
22	Tune into your body clock
24	Beat the winter chills
26	Stay safe in the sun
28	Get to grips with hay fever
30	Speak up for a better internet
32	Make money your friend

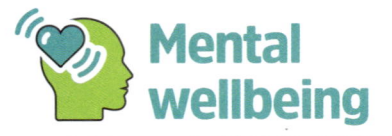

Mental wellbeing

36	Learn to cope with change
38	How to love who you are
42	Feel more confident
44	The power of positive thinking
46	Fill yourself with joy
48	The joy of colour
50	Make a colourful wind spinner
52	Celebrate the small stuff
54	Value your achievements
56	Stop caring what others think
58	The benefits of helping others
60	It's good to ask for help
62	Open your mind

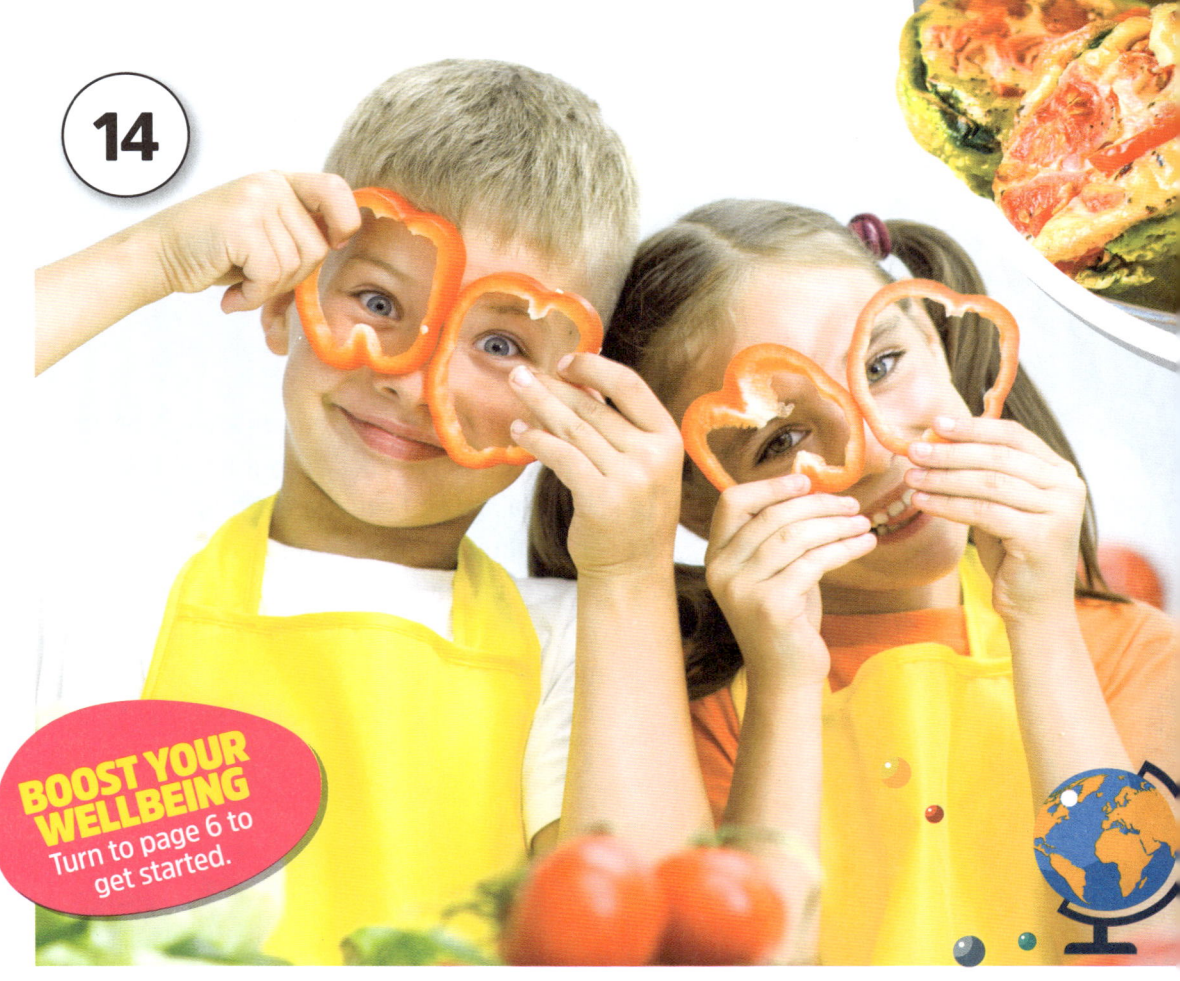

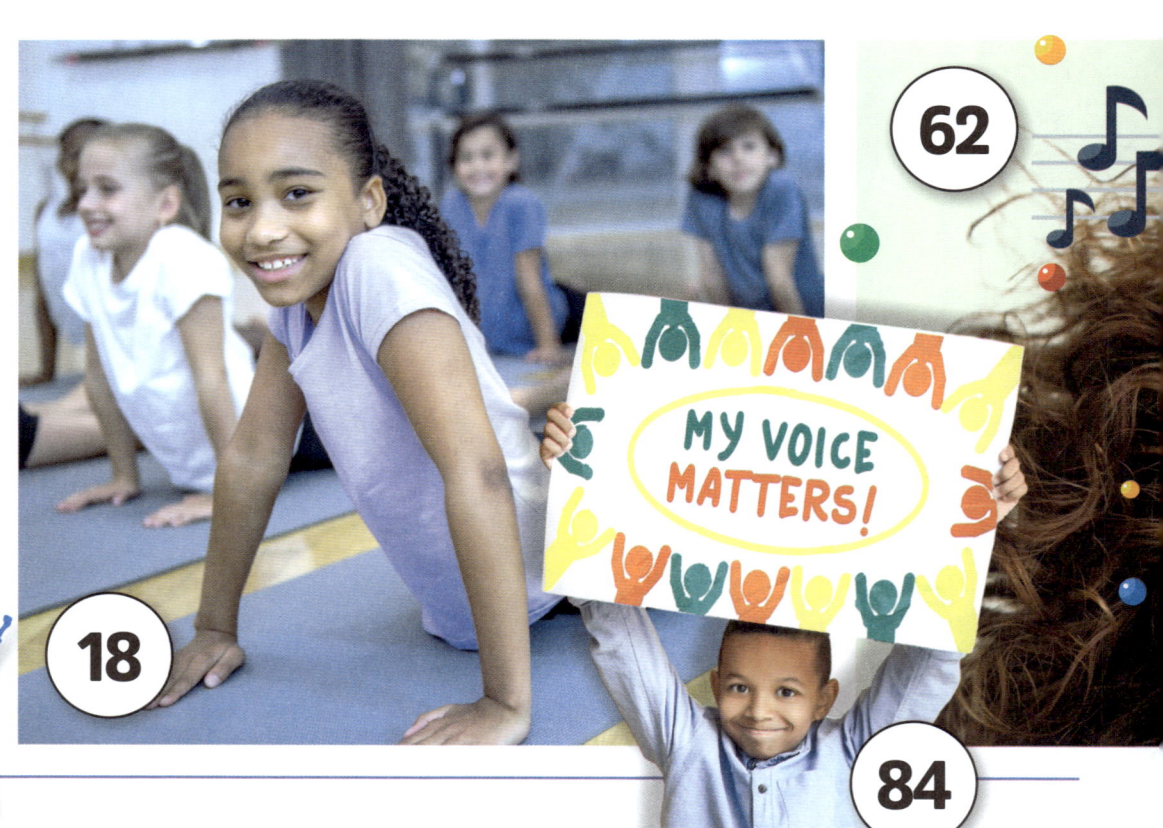

BOOST YOUR WELLBEING Turn to page 6 to get started.

MY VOICE MATTERS!

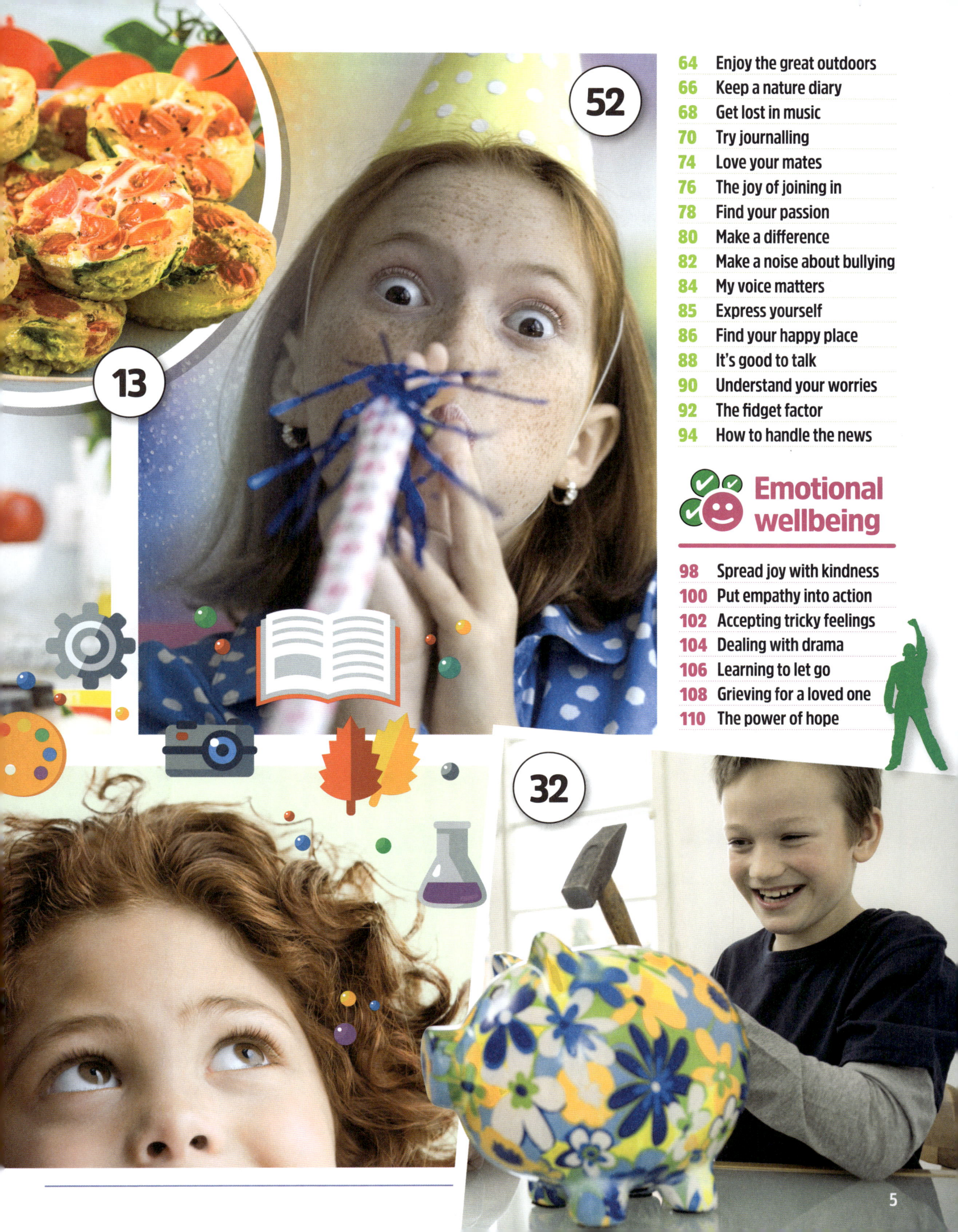

64	Enjoy the great outdoors
66	Keep a nature diary
68	Get lost in music
70	Try journalling
74	Love your mates
76	The joy of joining in
78	Find your passion
80	Make a difference
82	Make a noise about bullying
84	My voice matters
85	Express yourself
86	Find your happy place
88	It's good to talk
90	Understand your worries
92	The fidget factor
94	How to handle the news

Emotional wellbeing

98	Spread joy with kindness
100	Put empathy into action
102	Accepting tricky feelings
104	Dealing with drama
106	Learning to let go
108	Grieving for a loved one
110	The power of hope

Feel Good Guide

Boost your wellbeing

Learning to understand and accept yourself will help you as you grow.

Do you know how to unlock the magic of music, or that sport is a superpower? There are lots of ways you can boost your wellbeing, which means taking care of your physical, mental and emotional health. Physical health involves looking after your body. Caring for your mental health means understanding your feelings and learning how to manage them, while emotional wellbeing is feeling accepted and valued by yourself and other people.

According to the mental health charity Mind, wellbeing makes you feel positive about yourself and the world around you. It helps you understand yourself better so you can make good decisions and grow into the person you want to be. Feelings can change like the weather: some days you think you can climb a mountain while others you want to hide under your duvet, and this is okay.

Wellbeing doesn't mean being happy all the time, Mind explains, but it gives you the power to face challenges and cope with life's ups and downs.

Everyone is different and what works for your friends might not be the same for you. So *The Week Junior* has gathered lots of expert advice, facts and activities to improve your wellbeing in different ways. You can find out how food affects your emotions, the power of positive thinking and tips for opening up about your feelings. There's also practical advice like managing money and staying safe online. Plus we've included fun activities such as how to start a nature diary or make a colourful wind spinner. Wellbeing affects every part of your life, and finding ways to boost it now will help you as you grow.

Five steps to wellbeing

1 Connect. Connecting with people reminds us we're important and valued. This could be listening to others or speaking up if you see someone struggling.

2 Be active. Regular exercise makes you feel more positive. You don't have to be superfit: team sports and bike rides with friends all count.

3 Take notice. Being aware of what's going on around you helps you understand yourself better. Try keeping a journal of things you're grateful for.

4 Keep learning. Starting a new hobby or reading different books builds confidence and makes you feel closer to other people.

5 Give to others. Even small acts of kindness make a big difference, like saying thank you more often or volunteering at your school.

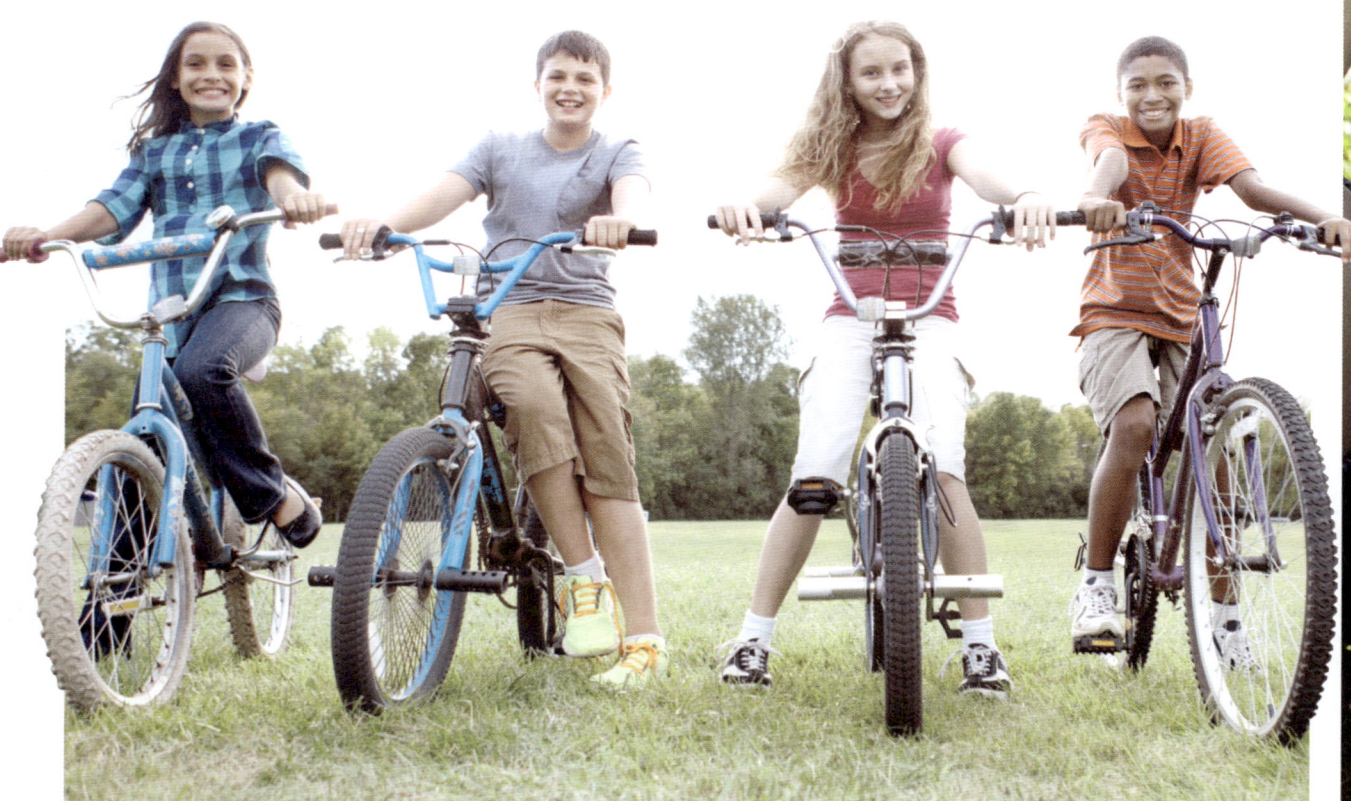

Boost your wellbeing

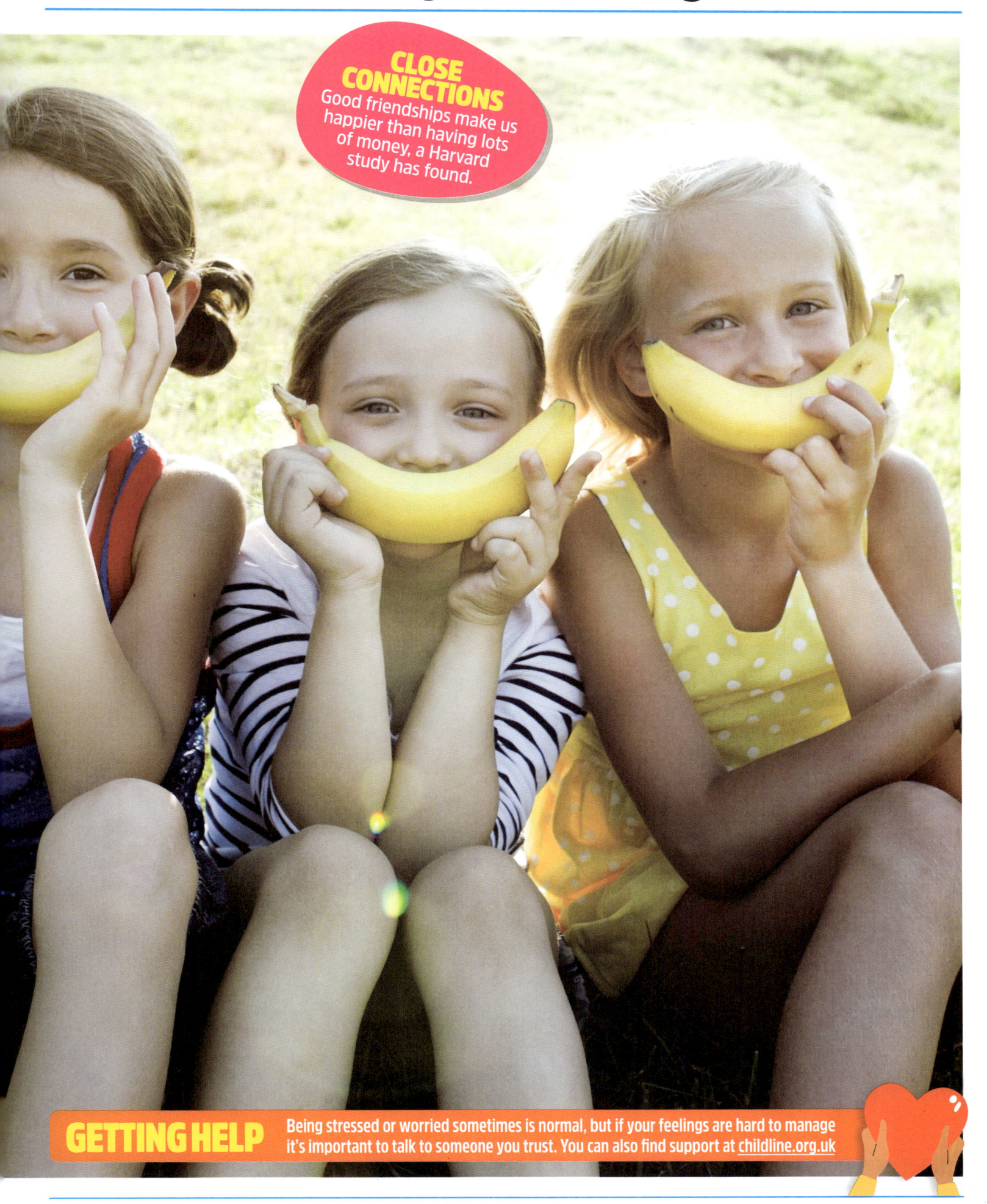

CLOSE CONNECTIONS
Good friendships make us happier than having lots of money, a Harvard study has found.

GETTING HELP Being stressed or worried sometimes is normal, but if your feelings are hard to manage it's important to talk to someone you trust. You can also find support at childline.org.uk

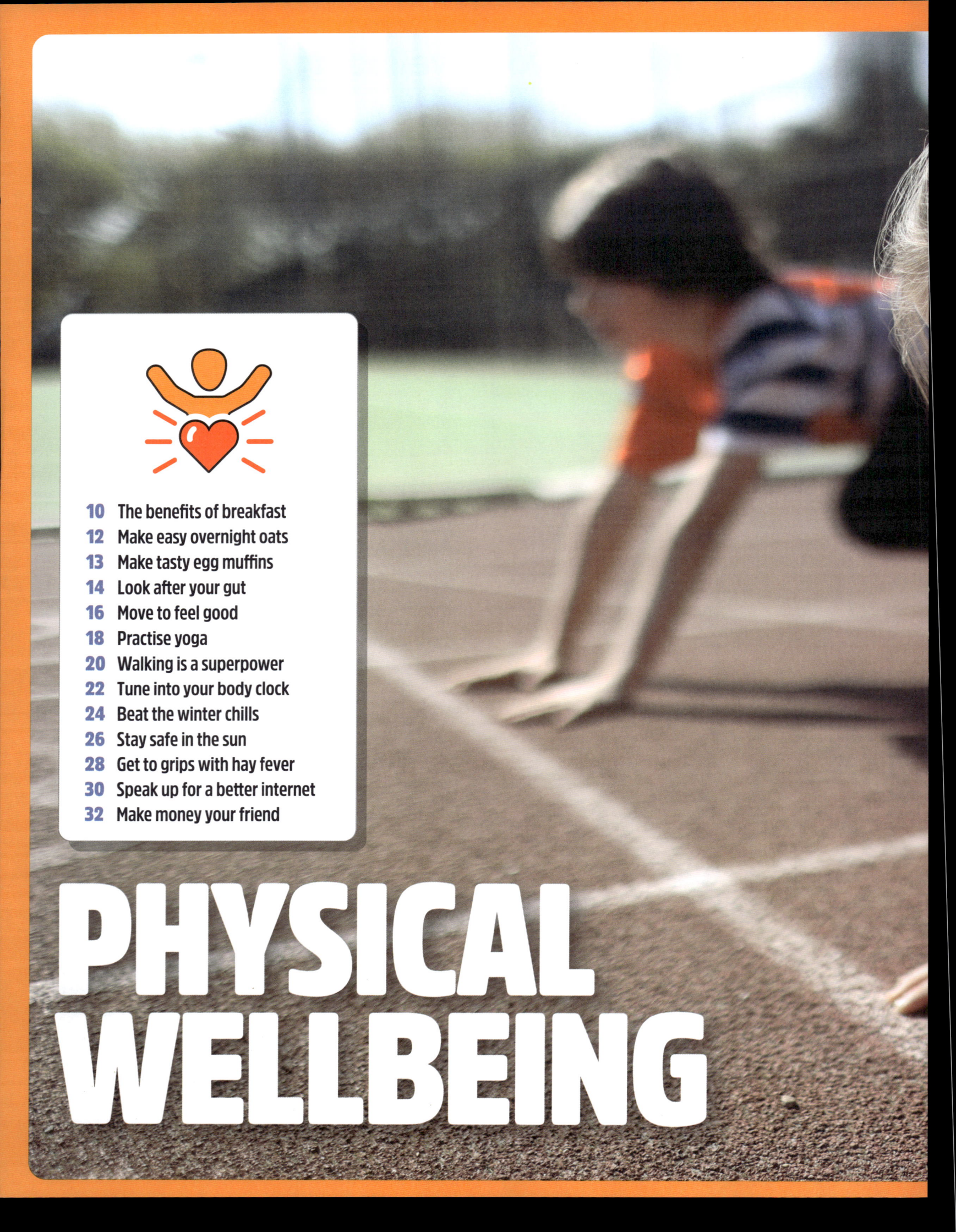

10   The benefits of breakfast
12   Make easy overnight oats
13   Make tasty egg muffins
14   Look after your gut
16   Move to feel good
18   Practise yoga
20   Walking is a superpower
22   Tune into your body clock
24   Beat the winter chills
26   Stay safe in the sun
28   Get to grips with hay fever
30   Speak up for a better internet
32   Make money your friend

PHYSICAL WELLBEING

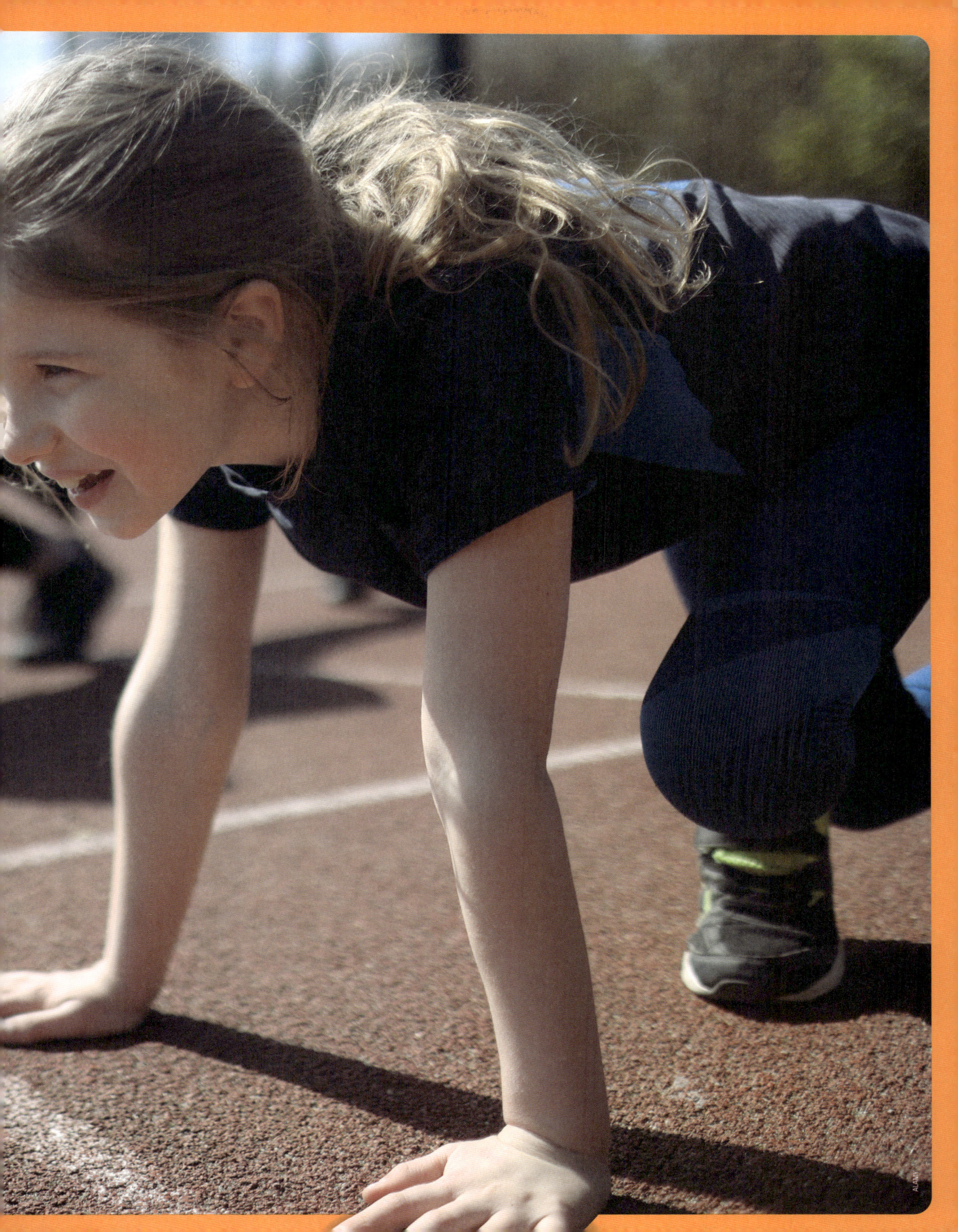

Physical wellbeing

The benefits of breakfast
Starting your day with a healthy meal boosts your focus and energy.

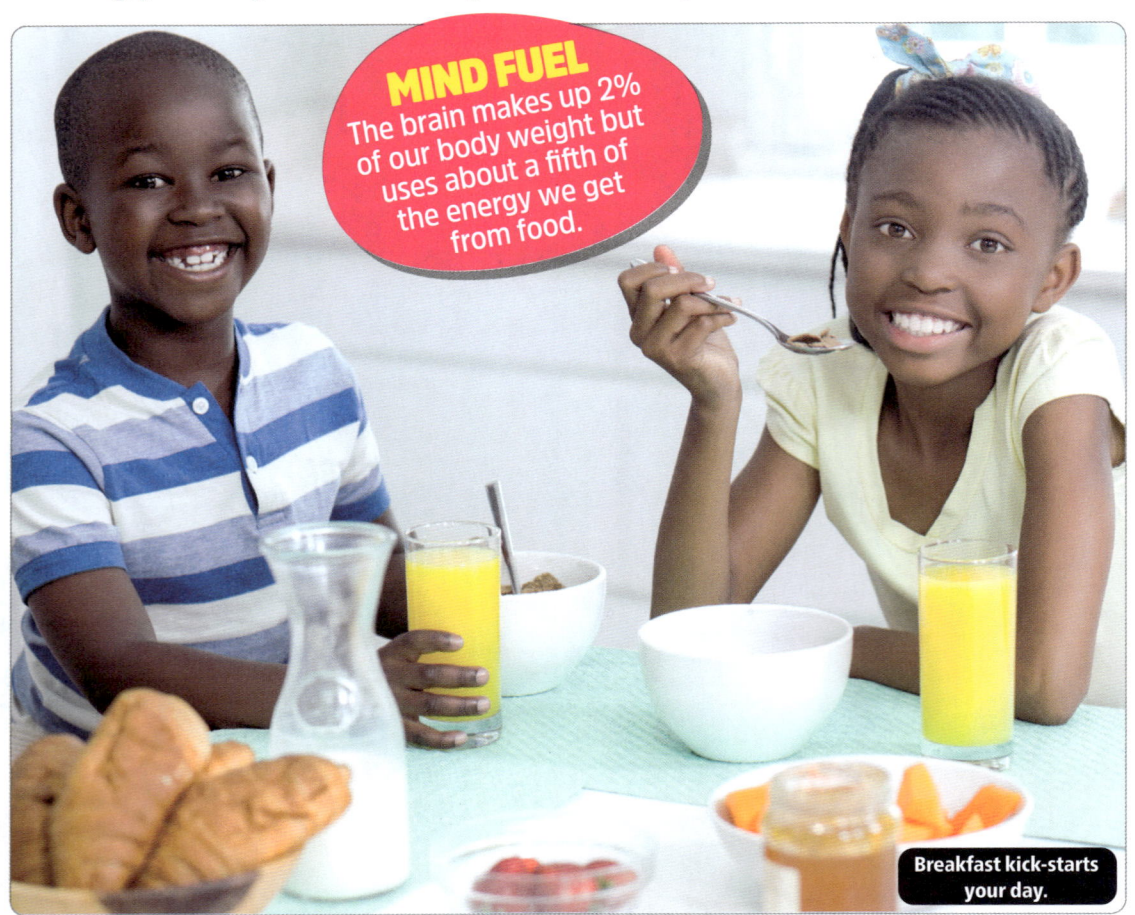

MIND FUEL
The brain makes up 2% of our body weight but uses about a fifth of the energy we get from food.

Breakfast kick-starts your day.

Why bother with breakfast?
Have you ever missed breakfast and spent the morning feeling sluggish and struggling to focus on things? Starting your day with a healthy, balanced meal is easy and it's great for your wellbeing, too.

Breakfast is a very important meal because it gives your energy a boost. It also provides the nutrients (important chemicals that your body uses), including vitamins, that your body needs to grow and work properly. Magic Breakfast is a charity that provides breakfasts to 200,000 children in England and Scotland. It says that eating a healthy meal before school makes it easier to focus and concentrate in lessons, and also helps you control your emotions so you're less likely to feel stressed or upset.

Breakfast for your brain
There are lots of studies that show the benefits breakfast has on your attention, memory and organising skills. This is because breakfast fuels your body and feeds your brain.

Smoothies are quick and easy.

When you wake up in the morning, you may not have eaten for 10 hours, which means your glucose levels will be low. Glucose is a type of sugar that comes from carbohydrates, which are found in bread, fruit, milk, nuts, seeds and beans. Scientists say our brains rely almost entirely on glucose for energy, so if you don't eat a healthy breakfast you may struggle to focus during the day.

Make time for breakfast
Chef and restaurant owner Jamie Oliver says, "Breakfast is so important because it kick-starts your day the right way." If you find yourself rushing in the mornings, try to make time to eat by getting up 10 minutes earlier. Oliver recommends filling up with a mixture of different foods in one dish so you're less likely to be tempted by sugary snacks before lunch. "Low or no-added sugar cereal or muesli is a good choice, as well as porridge with seasonal fruit and nuts, or home-made blueberry pancakes," he says. If you are short of time, Oliver suggests blitzing up some fruit and veg with yoghurt and oats for a quick smoothie.

Super scrambled eggs
Mix two eggs and a splash of milk together in a bowl. With help from an adult, melt some butter or margarine in a frying pan and add the egg mixture. Stir for a minute or so over a medium heat until the eggs are firm. Add extra flavour with a small pinch of dried chilli or mixed herbs. Serve on a slice of wholemeal toast with tomatoes.

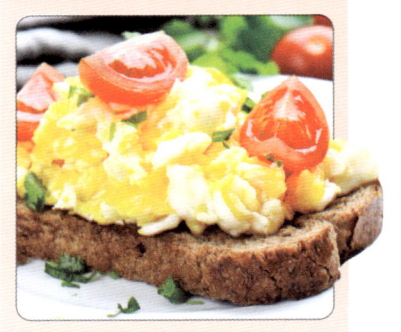

"Breakfast makes me feel energised"

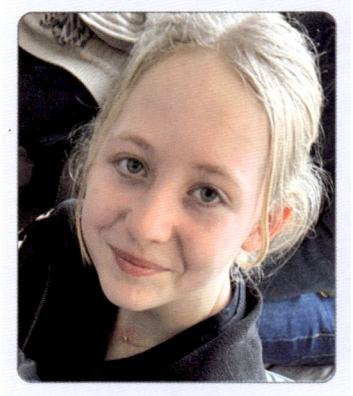

"I like fruit and fibre cereal for breakfast because it's easy to eat and I love the bits of dried banana. On weekends I sometimes have squashed avocado on toast. It helps me to feel energised."
Annie, aged 12

10

The benefits of breakfast

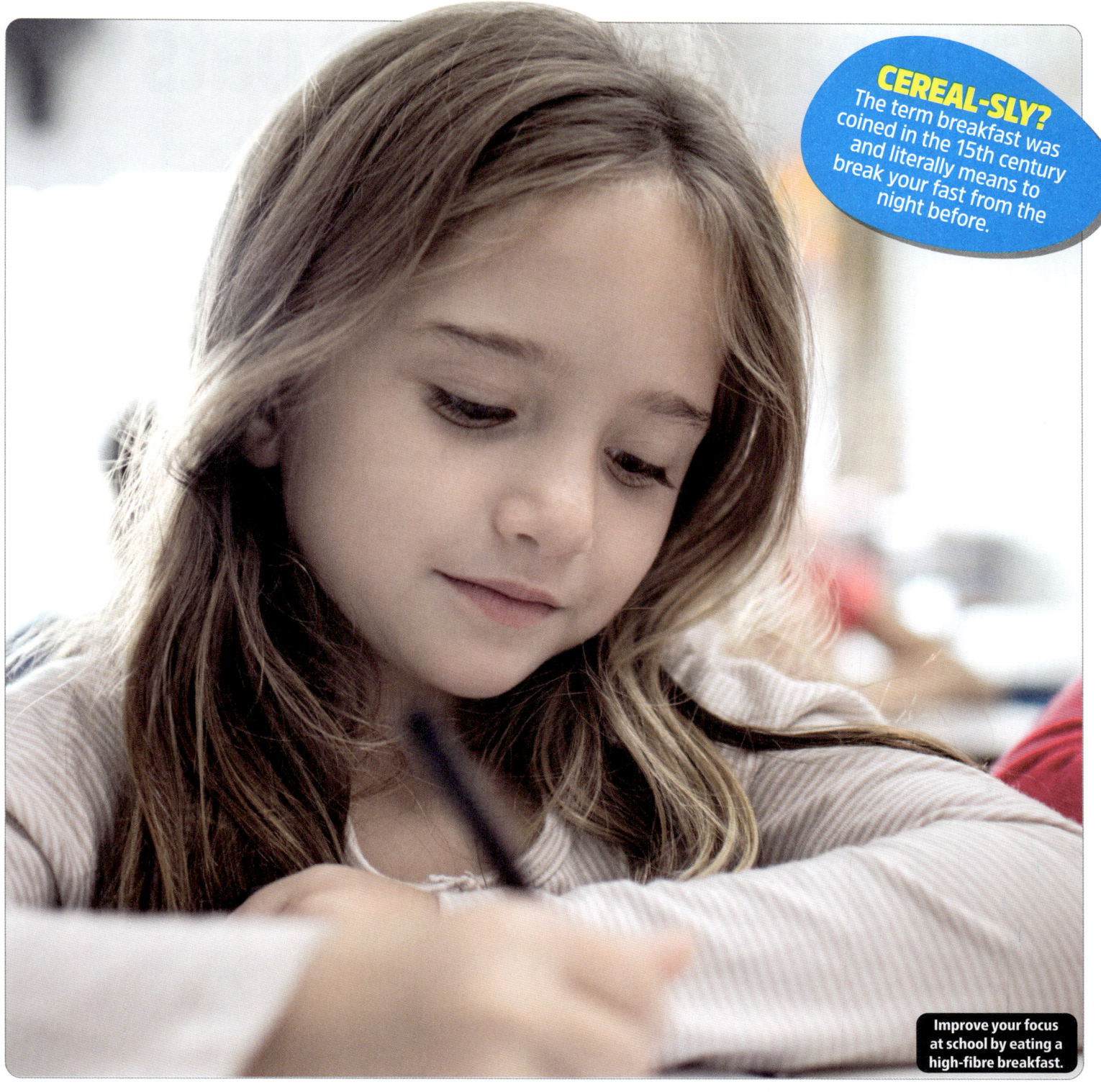

CEREAL-SLY? The term breakfast was coined in the 15th century and literally means to break your fast from the night before.

Improve your focus at school by eating a high-fibre breakfast.

Write down five healthy breakfast ideas to try:
_____
_____
_____
_____
_____

11

Physical wellbeing

Make easy overnight oats

What you need
- 40g (1.5oz) **porridge oats**
- Sprinkle of cinnamon
- 100ml (3.5fl oz) **milk**
- 1 tsp runny honey or maple syrup
- Half an apple

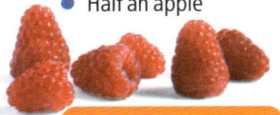

TOP TIP
Experiment with ingredients and flavours. Try mixing raspberries with coconut milk or banana with almond milk.

On school mornings it can be hard to find time to make a proper breakfast. This recipe, however, is prepared the night before, so breakfast is ready as soon as you get up. Overnight oats are a no-cook type of porridge – instead of cooking the oats on the hob, you soak them in milk for a few hours. This allows the grains to soak up the liquid and softens them enough so you can eat them uncooked. Hey presto! You have a healthy and delicious dish waiting for you in the fridge in the morning. This recipe makes one portion – multiply the ingredients for more people.

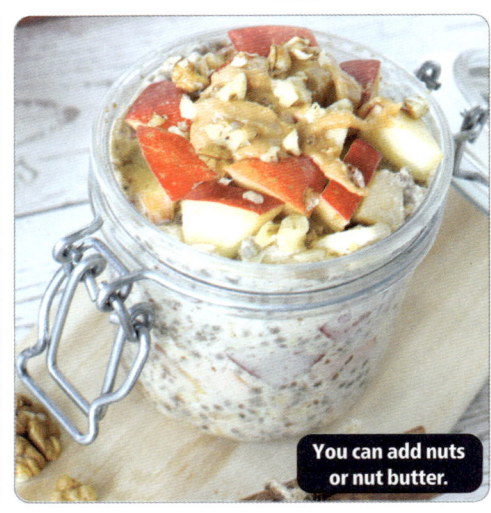

You can add nuts or nut butter.

1 Measure out the oats into a bowl and add a little cinnamon. Next, pour in the milk, drizzle in the honey and mix it up well.

2 Chop up the apple into small bite-sized pieces and scatter them on top of the oat mix.

3 Cover the mixture and put it in the fridge to rest overnight.

4 The next morning, uncover and enjoy. If you like, you can add a dollop of yoghurt or mix in some seeds or dried fruit, such as raisins.

Allergy information
Ingredients in **bold** are allergens. Allergens are substances that can cause allergic reactions in some people. If you have a food allergy, carefully check the items listed. You can find more information at tinyurl.com/TWJ-allergy

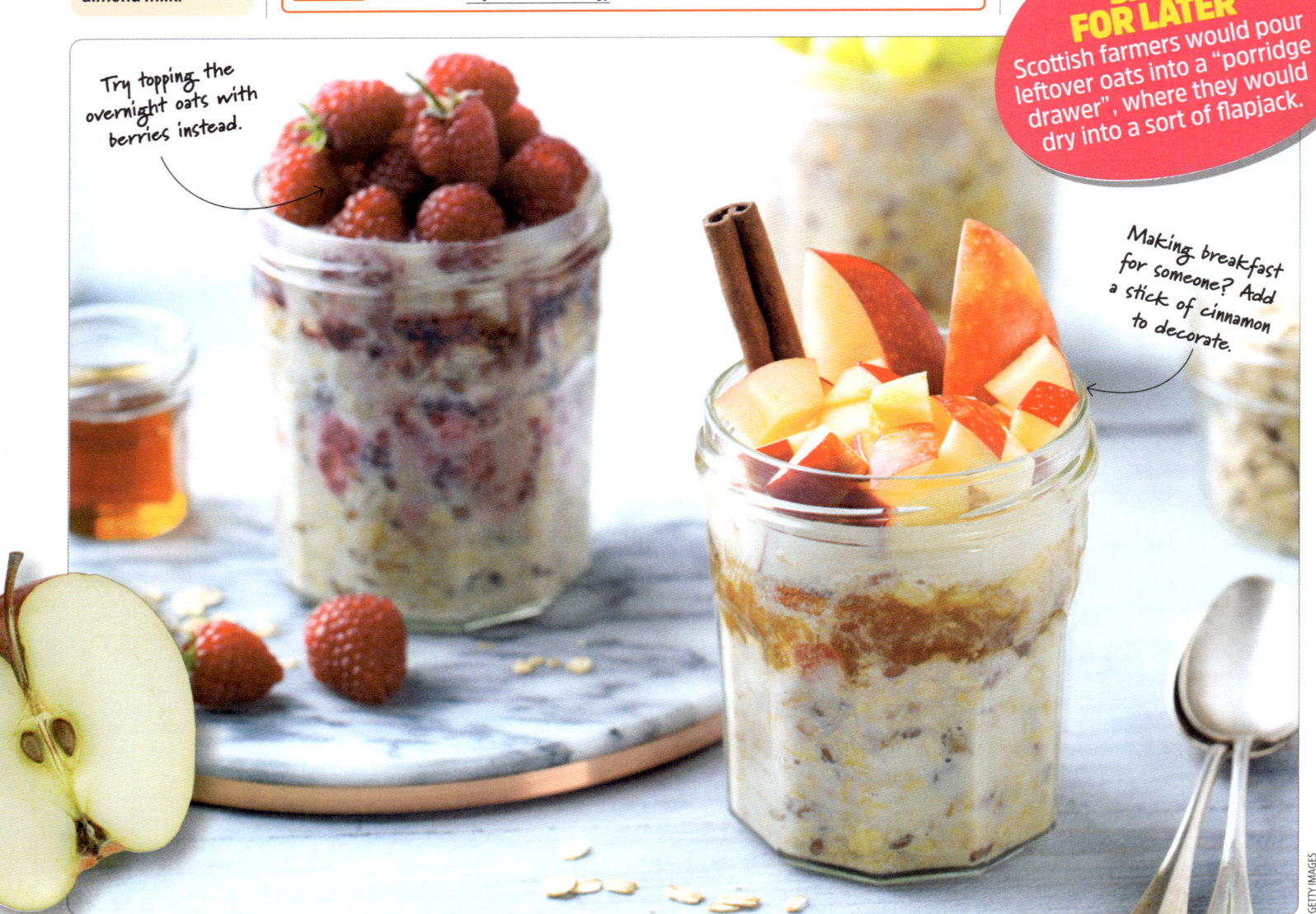

SAVE FOR LATER
Scottish farmers would pour leftover oats into a "porridge drawer", where they would dry into a sort of flapjack.

Try topping the overnight oats with berries instead.

Making breakfast for someone? Add a stick of cinnamon to decorate.

How to
Make tasty egg muffins

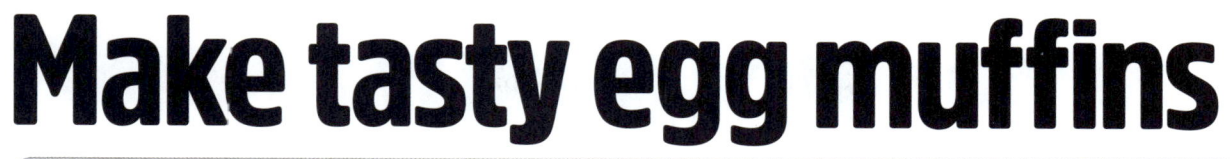

WARNING! Ask an adult to help you with the hot pan and oven.

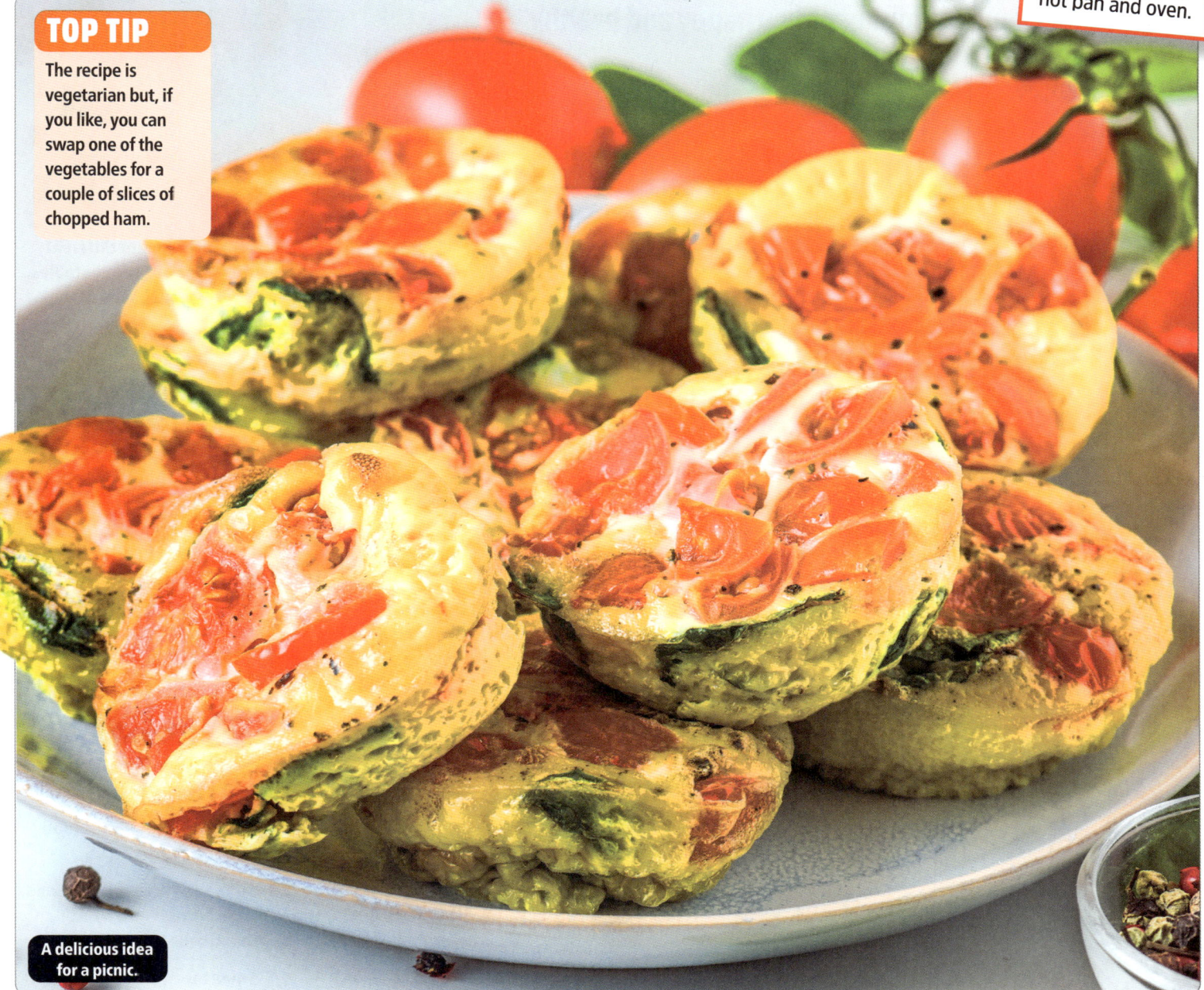

TOP TIP
The recipe is vegetarian but, if you like, you can swap one of the vegetables for a couple of slices of chopped ham.

A delicious idea for a picnic.

If you thought muffins had to be sweet, think again. These savoury treats are perfect for a picnic – or a breakfast that you can make in advance. The recipe is enough to make eight muffins in a muffin tin. If you don't have one of these, you can use silicone or paper muffin cases – but oil them well to stop the egg from sticking. If you haven't got all the vegetables, swap them for others that you like.

What you need
- 1 tbsp oil (oil spray works well)
- 150g (5oz) courgette, finely chopped or grated
- 2 tomatoes, finely chopped
- 2 spring onions, sliced
- 6 large **eggs**
- 1 tbsp **milk**
- Paprika (optional)
- 50g (2oz) **Cheddar cheese**, grated
- 8-hole muffin tin
- Pastry brush
- Frying pan
- Mixing bowl
- Chopping board

1 Heat the oven to 200°C/180°C Fan/400°F/Gas mark 6. Brush half the oil into the muffin tin or cases, or give each a generous spray of oil.

2 Heat the rest of the oil in a frying pan and add the chopped courgettes, tomatoes and spring onions. Stir fry for five minutes, then put them aside to cool.

3 Crack the eggs into your bowl with the milk, paprika and half the cheese and whisk it all up. Fold in the cooked vegetables.

4 Pour the egg mixture carefully and evenly into the muffin tin holes and top each with the remaining grated cheese.

5 Bake for 15–17 minutes or until they're golden brown and cooked through. Eat them warm or cold (they will keep in the fridge for three days).

Physical wellbeing

Look after your gut
Taking care of your tummy keeps you happy and healthy.

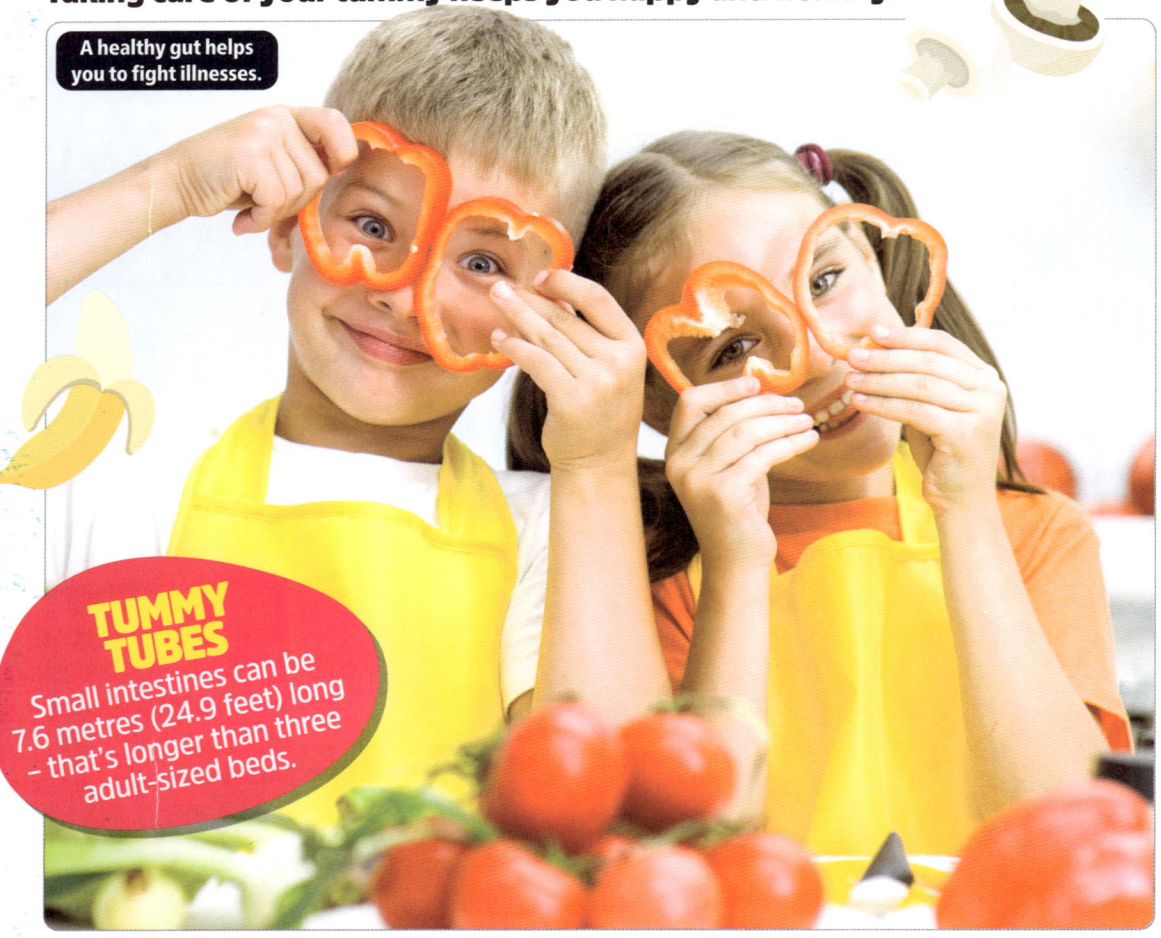

A healthy gut helps you to fight illnesses.

TUMMY TUBES
Small intestines can be 7.6 metres (24.9 feet) long – that's longer than three adult-sized beds.

Eat the rainbow

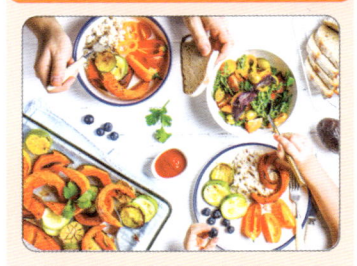

Eating a rainbow of different-coloured fruits and vegetables gives your body many of the substances you need to live and grow. Choose red food like strawberries; orange food such as carrots; green like broccoli; blue and purple blueberries and white, such as mushrooms.

How you digest food

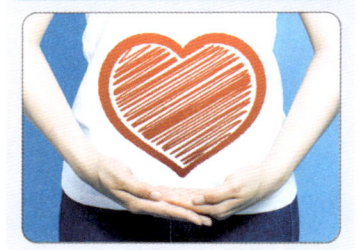

- **Mouth** – chewing softens food so it can be swallowed.
- **Oesophagus** – pushes food into the stomach.
- **Stomach** – breaks down food and churns it into a thick liquid called chyme.
- **Small intestine** – breaks food down into chemicals that the body can use.
- **Large intestine** – remaining food is digested or turned into solid waste (poo) and passes out of the body.

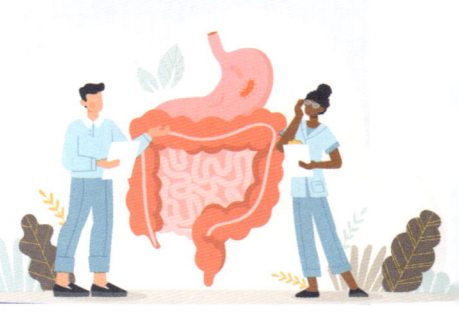

Have you ever felt butterflies in your tummy when you're nervous or excited? This is because there is a close connection between your gut and your brain. Looking after your gut is not only good for your health, it can help to manage emotions too.

What is your gut?
Your digestive system, or gut, includes your mouth, oesophagus (food pipe), stomach and intestines. It is where your body digests food, absorbs energy and nutrients (substances that we need to live and grow) and gets rid of waste. Living inside your gut are trillions of bacteria and other microbes (tiny, simple forms of life) that help break down the food you eat.

How is a healthy gut good for you?
You have around 200 types of microbe in your gut. "They have thousands of responsibilities and are connected to pretty much every function of your body," says Dr Megan Rossi, a scientist and author. Microbes' jobs include producing vitamins and hormones (chemicals) to keep your body working properly, and letting your brain know when you're hungry. Healthy microbes boost your energy and strengthen your immune system, which helps your body fight illnesses. They are also involved in helping your brain manage emotions and deal with stress. However, your gut "can only look after you if you look after it," says Rossi.

Water helps your gut.

Looking after yourself
Eating lots of different foods from plants keeps the microbes in your gut happy, Rossi explains. These foods include fruit, vegetables, beans and pulses (lentils, chickpeas), as well as wholemeal bread and rice. Rossi recommends chewing each mouthful 10 to 15 times, depending on the food, so your saliva can start breaking it down. "In our mouths is where digestion begins," Rossi says. You can take care of your gut by getting plenty of exercise to help move the muscles that push the food through your digestive system, too. Drinking water regularly also helps your body get rid of waste.

14

Look after your gut

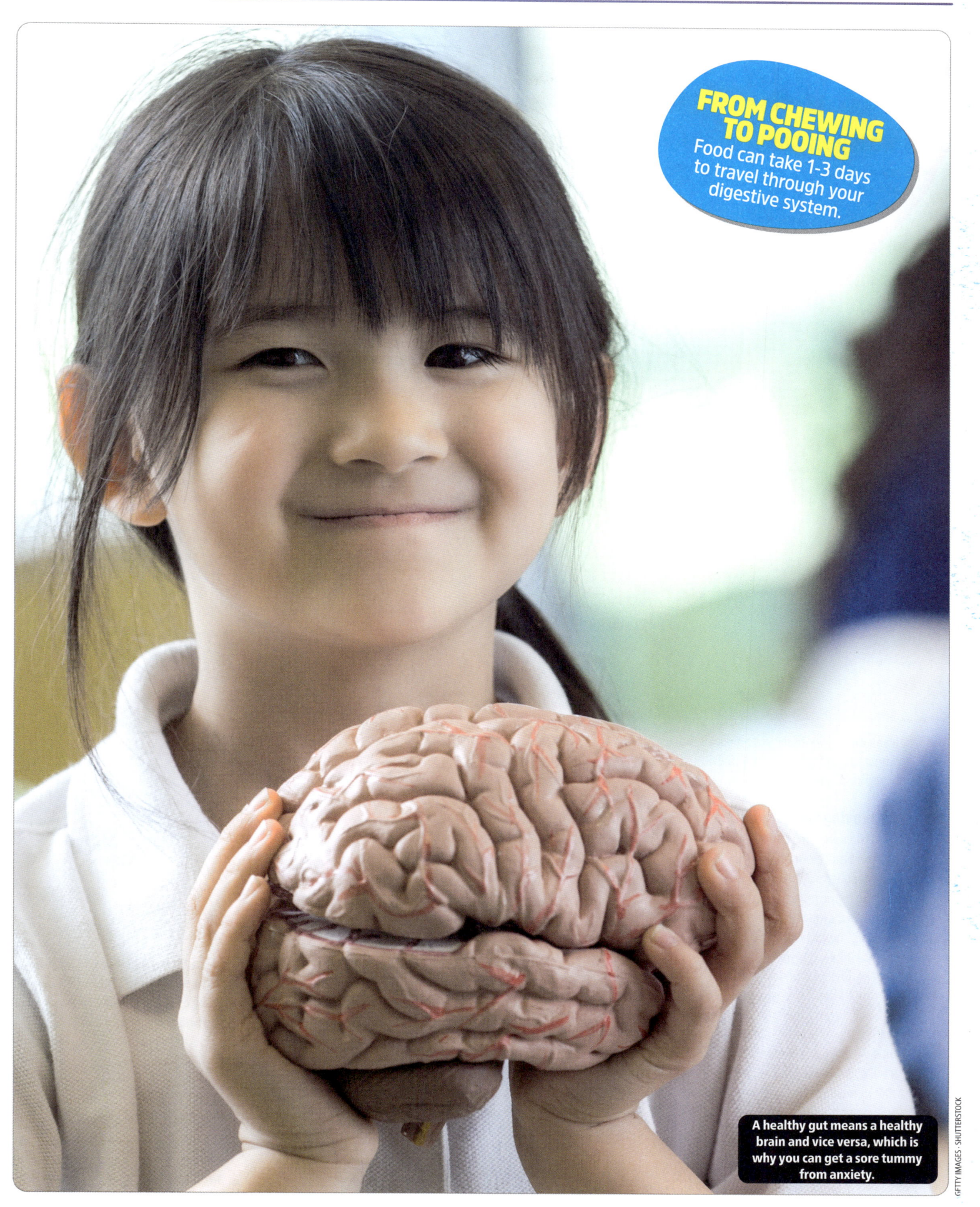

FROM CHEWING TO POOING
Food can take 1-3 days to travel through your digestive system.

A healthy gut means a healthy brain and vice versa, which is why you can get a sore tummy from anxiety.

15

Physical wellbeing

Move to feel good

Enjoy what your body can do for your mood and your mind.

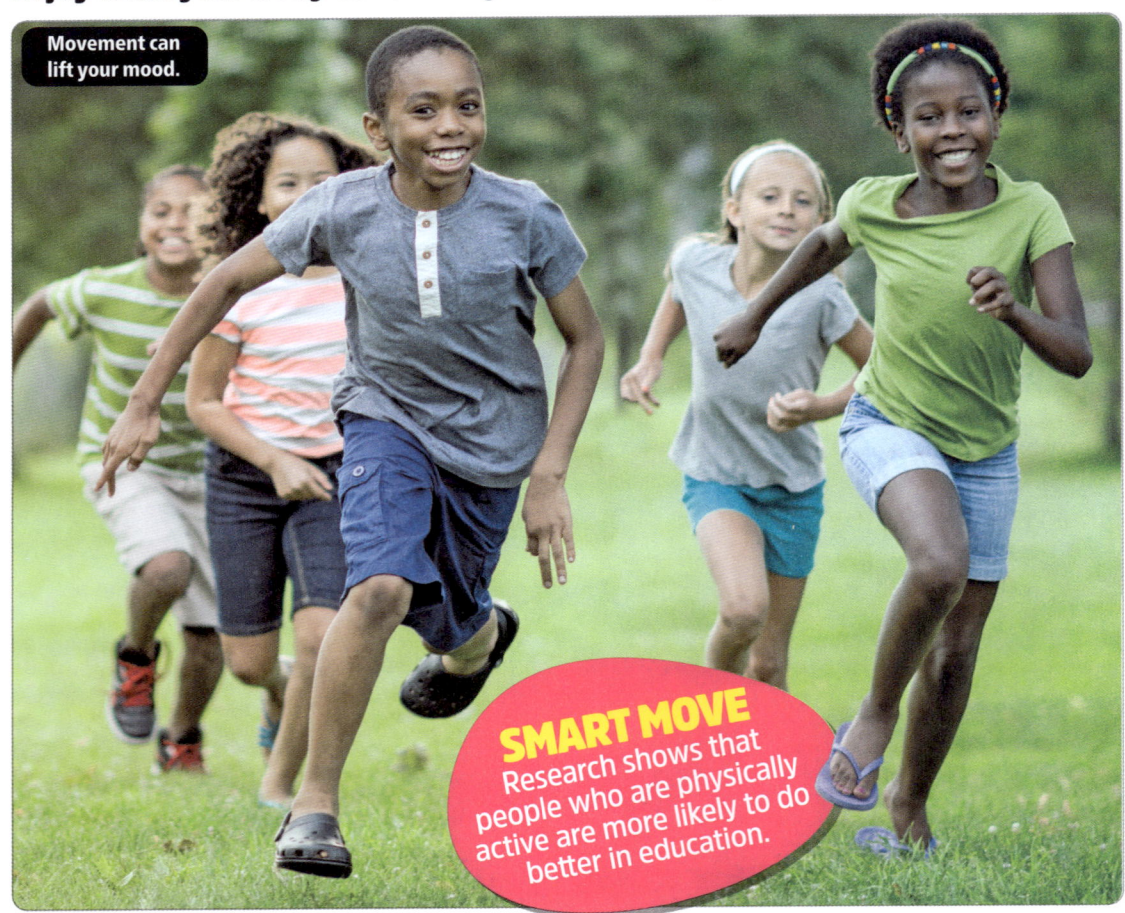

Movement can lift your mood.

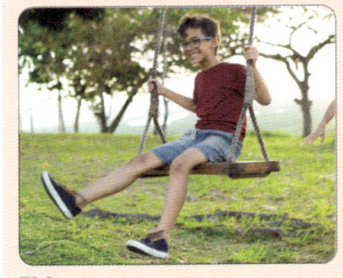

SMART MOVE
Research shows that people who are physically active are more likely to do better in education.

Try what feels good

Things you can try:
- Swimming
- Ball games
- Throwing a Frisbee
- Trampolining
- Playing in the park
- Walking the dog
- Cycling
- Skipping
- Dancing
- Gardening

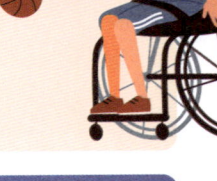

"I like to jump about and dance"

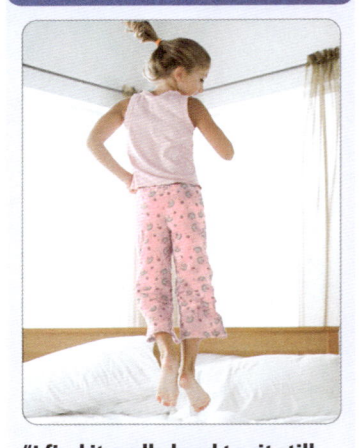

When you move your body, your muscles, bones, mind and heart all feel the benefits – physical activity makes you happy and strong from the inside out.

Why does moving feel so good?
The mind and the body are connected, so when we are active and move our bodies, our minds usually feel better. This is because movement reduces the levels of stress hormones (chemicals made by the body) and boosts chemicals that make you feel happy. Lildonia Lawrence is a wellbeing coach. She says noticing your body's sensations can make you more aware of how your thoughts and feelings are affected. "Think of a time when you've ridden a bike down a hill and felt the wind against your face. Or when you make up a dance routine with your friend," says Lawrence.

Studies show that people who are active – anything that raises your energy levels and gets your heart pumping – feel happier and more confident. This can be useful if you're feeling anxious or sad.

Find activities you enjoy.

"When we feel unhappy, our body releases stress hormones," says Lawrence. "That's why parents or caregivers might say let's go for a walk, because it can help shift your energy."

Your body and your brain
Exercise also helps the brain to work better. Lawrence says when you feel fidgety or distracted, doing something active can release that energy. "Some schools walk laps of the playground in break time. Others start their classes with simple yoga and breathing. These help you to feel calm and focused," she explains.

Find what works for you
You don't need to play sport or go for long runs to enjoy the benefits of movement. Spend time outdoors, throw a Frisbee, play ballgames with friends, walk the dog or dance to music. These all make a positive difference. Lawrence suggests making a list of five types of movement that you enjoy. It doesn't matter what they are – the aim is to find out what feels good for you. Then, if you suddenly notice you are restless or anxious, you can turn to your list of what you enjoy and get going.

"I find it really hard to sit still, so when I've got lots of energy I like to jump about! Most nights before I go to bed I have a moment of dancing around the living room, it wears me out so I can go to sleep. I like playing football too. I even like to play when it's raining because running around makes me so happy."
Jazz, aged 12

Move to feel good

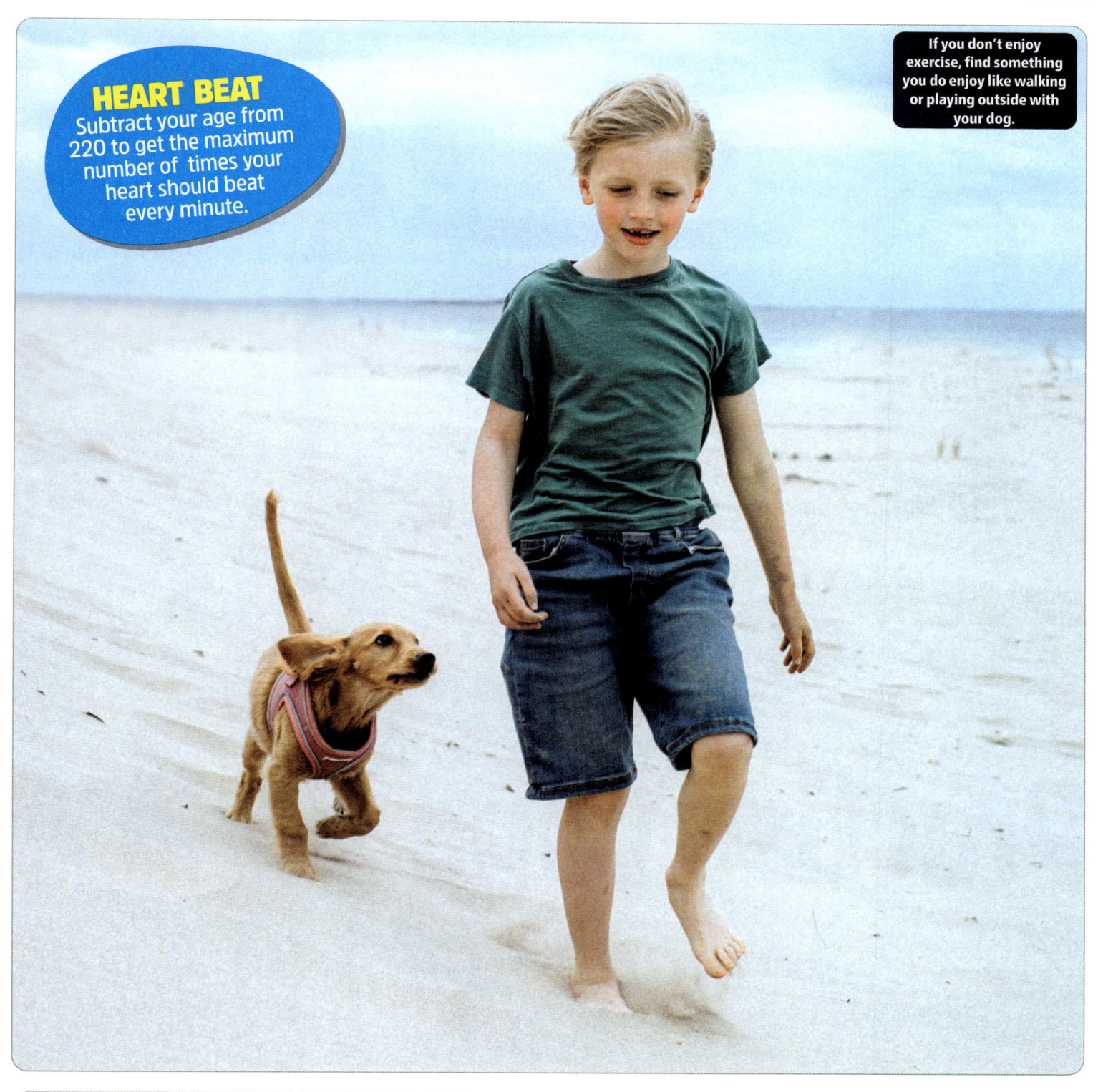

HEART BEAT
Subtract your age from 220 to get the maximum number of times your heart should beat every minute.

If you don't enjoy exercise, find something you do enjoy like walking or playing outside with your dog.

Make a list of five types of movement you enjoy:

Physical wellbeing

Yoga relaxes your body and mind.

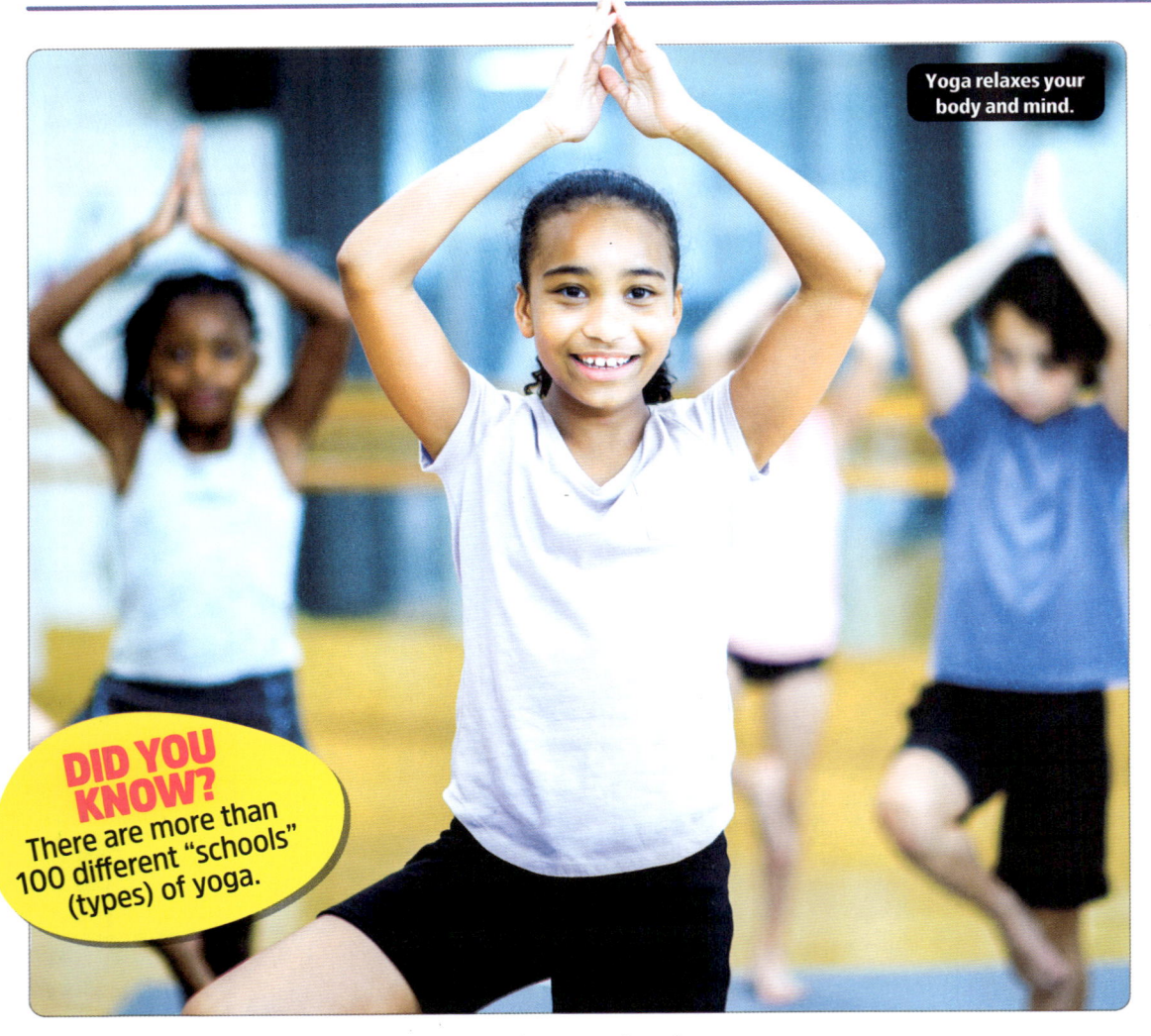

DID YOU KNOW? There are more than 100 different "schools" (types) of yoga.

Stretch, pose and boost your happiness when you…

Practise yoga

Have you ever performed the cat, cobra, cow or crocodile? Then you might have tried yoga. Yoga is a form of exercise that involves stretching and holding poses. The poses are often named after animals, such as butterfly, downward dog and dragon. There's also a tree pose – and even a "happy baby".

Yoga first developed in India around 5,000 years ago and is now popular all over the world. Millions of people of all ages and abilities do it every day to boost their health and wellbeing.

The poses might look easy but it takes practice to do them properly. It's a good idea to get expert advice too, to make sure you are doing them correctly. Practising yoga has many benefits. The stretches and poses work a range of muscles and help to build strength and flexibility. Yoga can also improve balance and concentration. It's also relaxing. Performing the poses and thinking carefully about your breathing at the same time gives your mind a new focus and helps you forget your worries. If you can't stand for too long or struggle with balance, then you could try seated yoga, which involves doing stretches and poses with a chair. A full yoga session can last from 10 minutes to an hour, but a class for a young beginner usually lasts about 20 to 30 minutes – enough to learn the basics.

Jen Hoe is a yoga instructor who visits schools to run workshops and teach young people about yoga and its benefits. "I love yoga and I love teaching youngsters about yoga," she says. "It's a fun way of moving and stretching your body that helps you feel happy and healthy. It's also a way of keeping our minds calm." With all these benefits on offer, it's a great exercise to try for the start of a new school year.

Everyone can try yoga.

ESSENTIAL YOGA POSES FOR BEGINNERS

Discover how to build strength, flexibility and mental wellbeing with this ancient form of movement

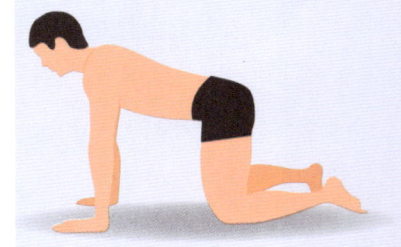

1 Cat/cow pose
Start on your hands and knees, with wrists under your shoulders and knees under your hips, lining up at 90-degree angles. When you breathe out, round your spine, pulling your head towards your nave. As you breathe in, turn your head towards the sky and open the chest, creating a curve in your spine. This is a great stretch for the back and hips.

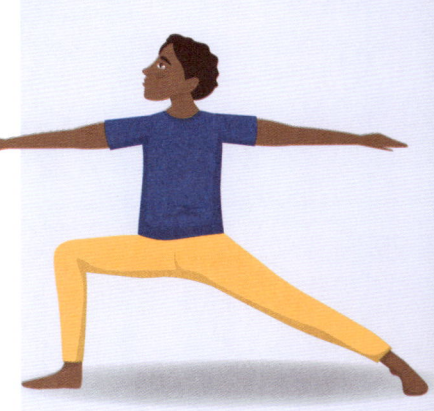

2 Warrior II pose
Stand with your feet wide apart. Start with your right foot and turn it 90 degrees to the right. Your left foot should turn about 45 degrees to the right. The heel of your right foot should be in line with the side arch of your left foot. Bend your knee towards the right foot so that your knee sits directly over your ankle, but keep your core centred between both feet. Your arms stretch out to both sides, and you look forward towards your right foot. Repeat on the left side.

Practise yoga

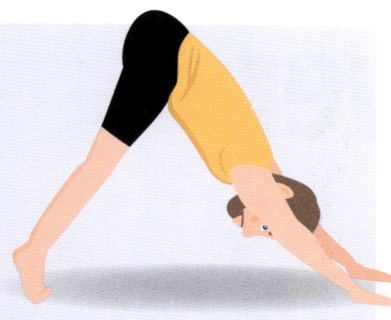

SMART MOVE
Yoga can improve your IQ according to research.

3 Downward-facing dog
Starting on all fours, with wrists under shoulders and knees under hips, lift your knees up and push your hips towards the sky. Your hands should be firm to the ground. Push your chest and head between your arms, and keep your core tight. You may have to bend your knees to start if your hamstrings are tight. You're aiming to create straight lines and form a triangle.

4 Standing forward bend
Start in a standing position, with feet firmly planted hip-width apart. Draw your spine to its full length, then bend forwards, hinging at the hips. With each breath try to relax the neck and shoulders. Your hands can hang, grasp your ankles or lightly touch the floor for support. Your knees should be bent as much as you need, and you can start to straighten them over time.

5 Child's pose
Kneel down and tip forward, bringing your arms in front of you, forehead to the floor and push your chest down. Keep your bottom pushing towards your heels and lengthen through your spine. Take deep breaths as you sink into the pose and hold. This can help to release tension in the body, as well as help your back to stay strong and flexible.

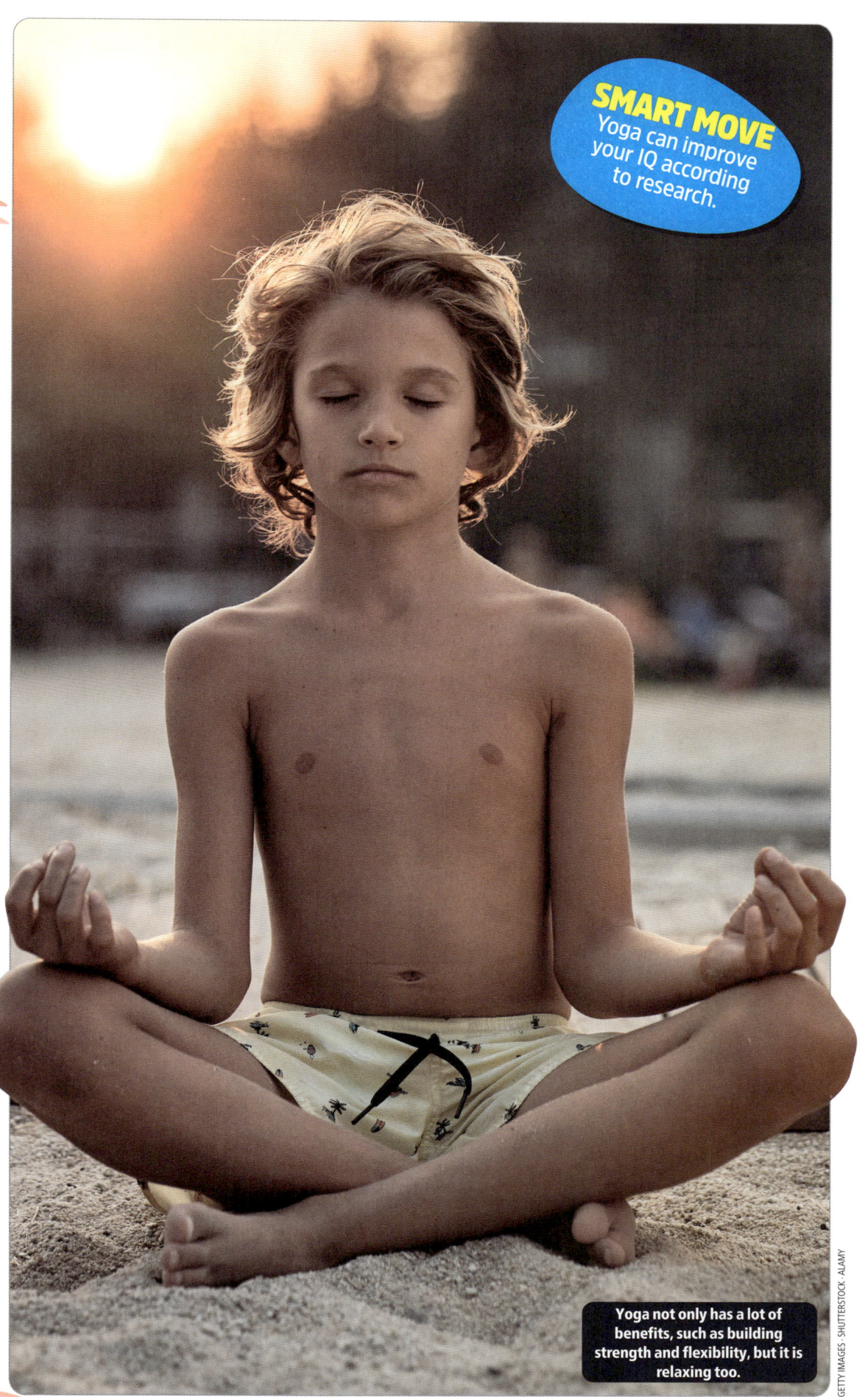

Yoga not only has a lot of benefits, such as building strength and flexibility, but it is relaxing too.

Physical wellbeing

Walking is a superpower

Experts say regular walks make us happier, healthier and brainier.

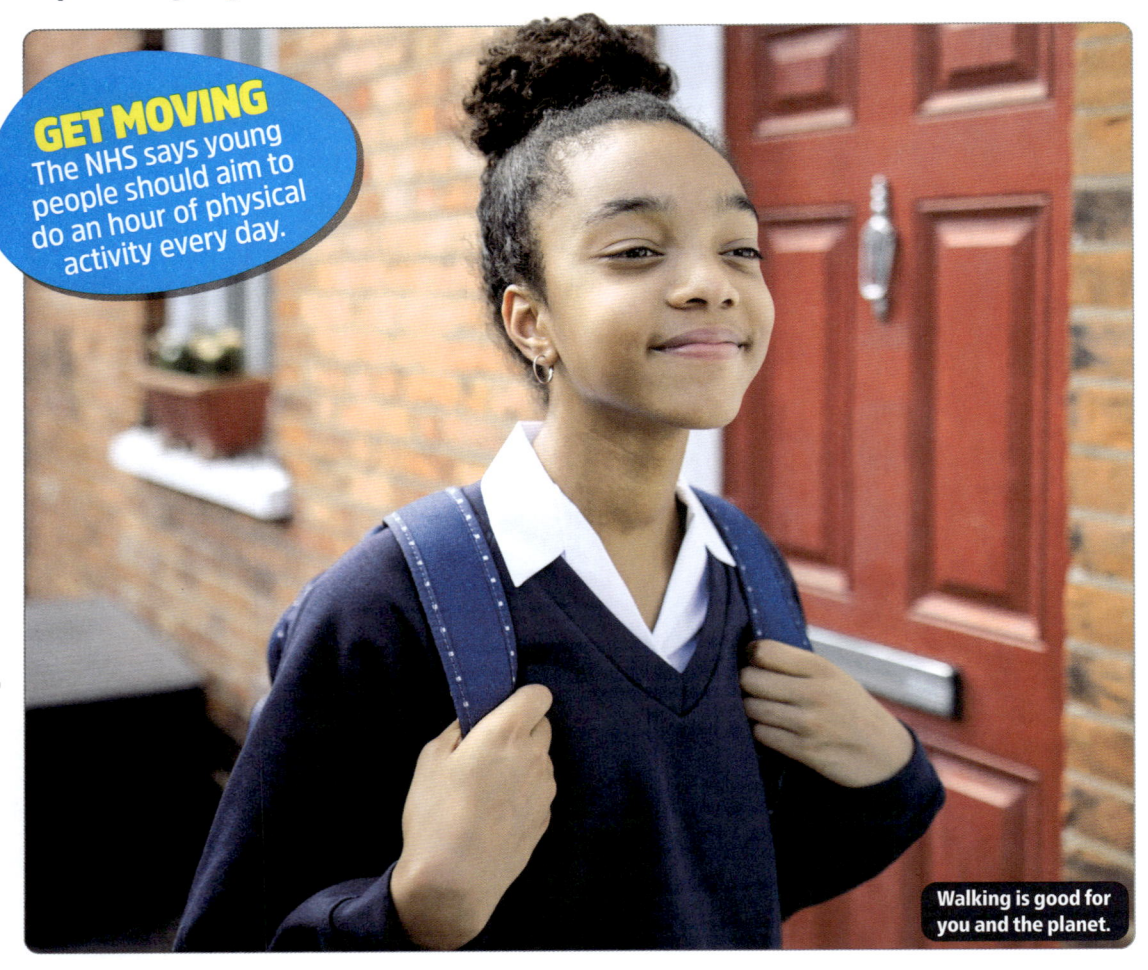

GET MOVING
The NHS says young people should aim to do an hour of physical activity every day.

Walking is good for you and the planet.

As well as being better for the environment, regular walking can boost your body and mind.

Why is walking good for you?
Have you ever noticed you have more energy after a walk? According to experts, walking isn't just good for your physical health, it can also clear your mind, sharpen your senses and lift your mood. In fact, scientist and author Shane O'Mara calls walking "one of the great, overlooked superpowers" because it makes your brain work harder. Making walks part of your daily routine means you can use this superpower more often.

Make the most of your walks
Walking frequently with friends or family is a great opportunity to catch up and talk about your day, including any friendship or homework worries you may have. *The Week Junior* reader Cai, who is eight, says, "I like walking to school because I often see friends on the way in and we get to chat about stuff, which is fun." If your journey takes you through fields or a park, you could make a game out of trying to spot a different bird or insect every day. Walking along pavements is a chance to practise road safety skills and get to know your neighbourhood better.

Cai likes to walk and talk.

What if you can't walk all the way to school?
Not everyone can get to school on foot but there are lots of ways to make walking or exercise part of your daily routine. If you catch a bus, try getting off a stop early and walking the rest of the way. Or if you arrive by car, ask your parents or carer to park further away. Fewer cars outside the school gates will also mean less pollution (harmful gases and chemicals) in the air, which is good for everybody and the planet too. A big part of fitting exercise into your everyday life is making it easy and fuss-free. "You don't need to bring anything other than comfy shoes and a rain jacket," says O'Mara.

Tips for a safe walk
- Always tell a parent or carer where you're going and what time you'll be home.
- Stick to busy and well-lit areas, especially during darker winter months.
- Carry some spare cash in case of emergencies.
- Try to avoid distractions like playing with your mobile phone or wearing headphones.

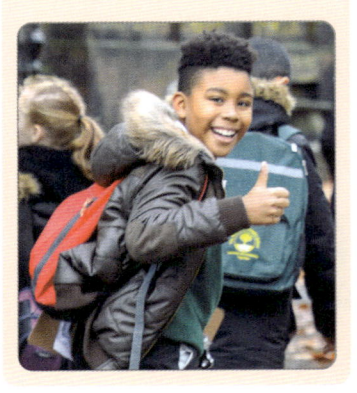

Keep a walk journal
The charity Living Streets suggests keeping a record of your walks by answering these questions – or you could come up with some of your own.

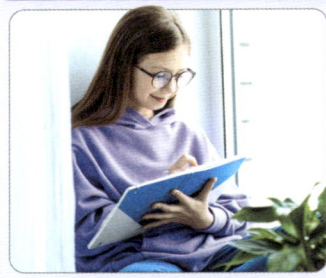

- Write three words about your walk.
- Sum up your walk with a quote (famous or made-up).
- If your walk was a song, what would it be?
- Who would you have liked to walk with you today?

Walking is a superpower

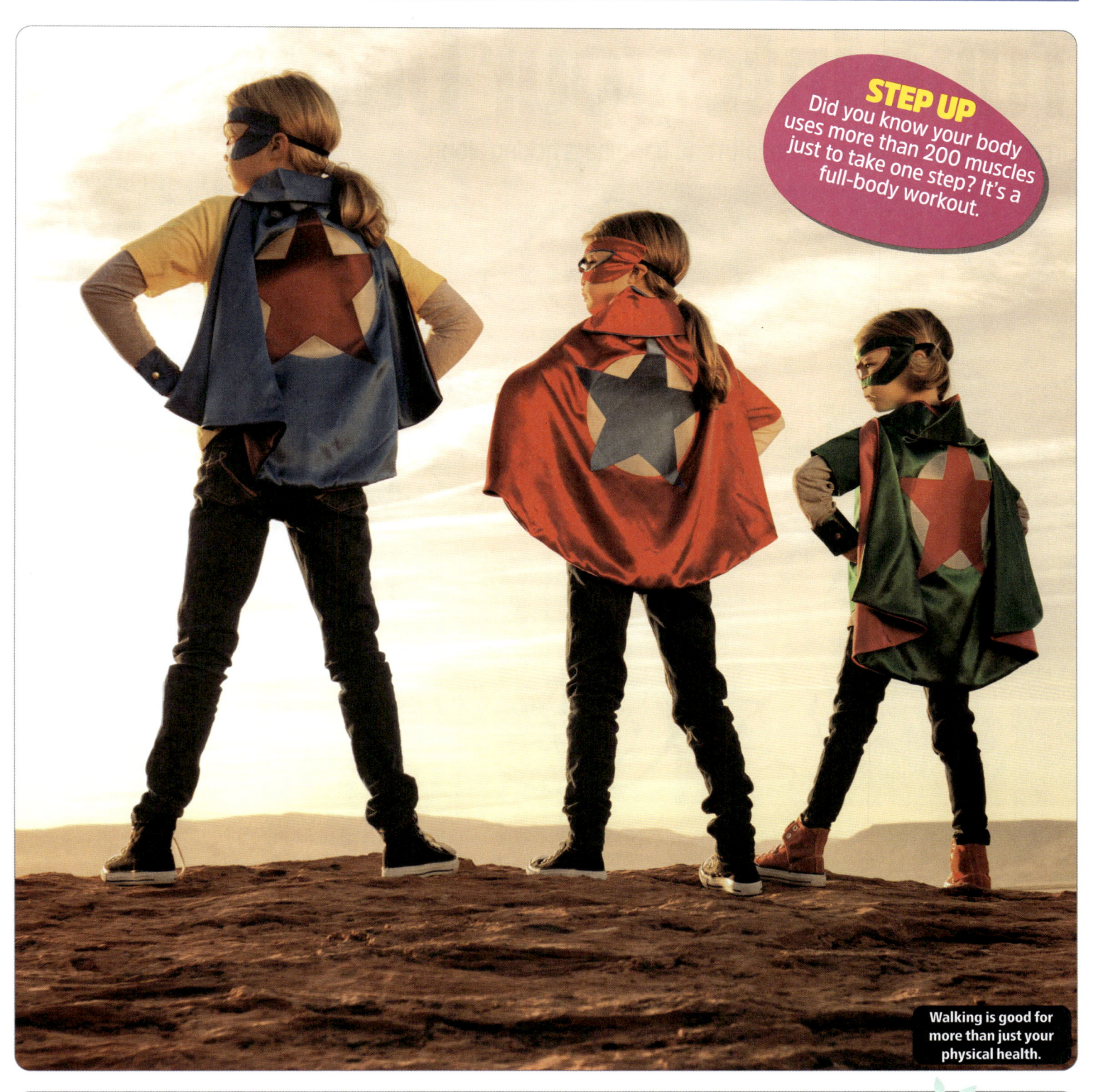

STEP UP
Did you know your body uses more than 200 muscles just to take one step? It's a full-body workout.

Walking is good for more than just your physical health.

Your walk journal:

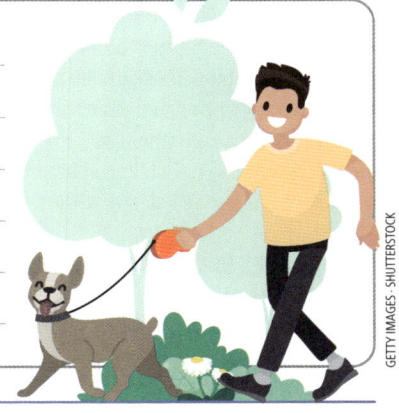

Physical wellbeing

Tune into your body clock

Circadian rhythms keep your health and happiness ticking along.

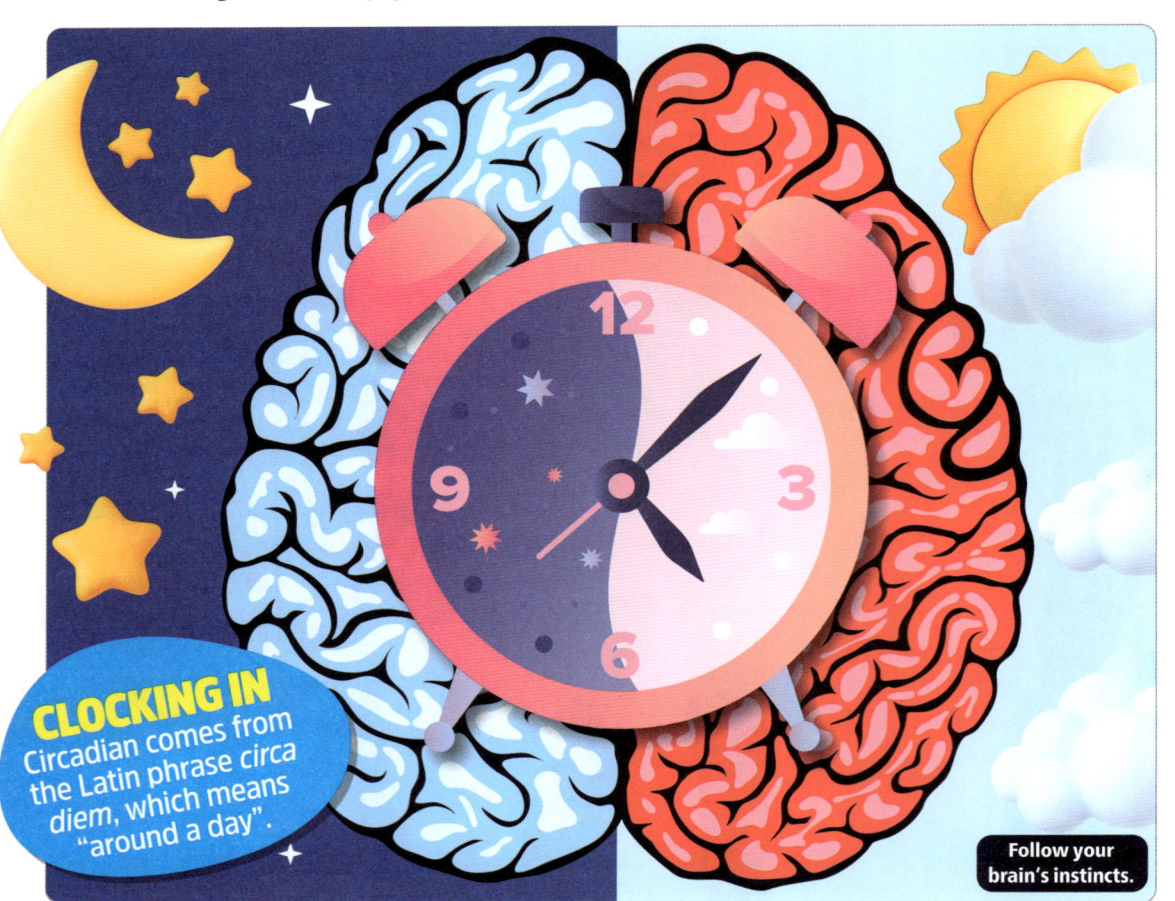

CLOCKING IN
Circadian comes from the Latin phrase *circa diem*, which means "around a day".

Follow your brain's instincts.

Tips for a healthy body clock

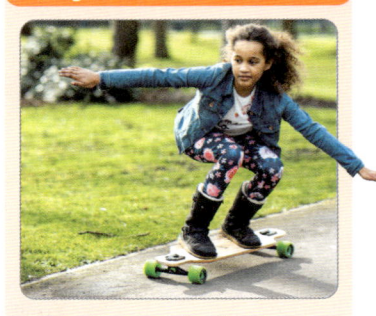

- Regular exercise helps you sleep better at night.
- Avoid eating sugary snacks or caffeine drinks before bedtime.
- Steer clear of screens before bed. Try reading a book or listening to music instead.

The circadian rhythm cycle

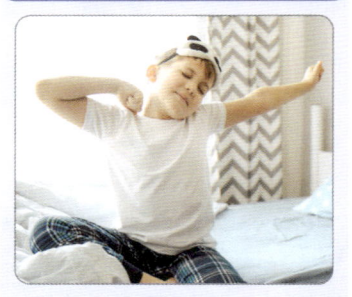

7.30am – your brain stops releasing a sleep hormone (chemical) called melatonin.

10am – your brain feels the most alert.

5pm – the best time to exercise.

7pm – your body temperature is at its highest.

9pm – melatonin is released to make you feel sleepy.

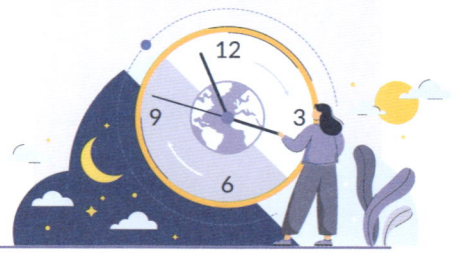

Have you wondered how your body knows when to wake up or why you need the loo less at night? Circadian rhythms use the sun to help your body to run on time.

What are circadian rhythms?
"Circadian rhythms" is another name for body clocks. They are controlled by a small part of the brain called the hypothalamus and they let the body know when to do things like eat, sleep and wee. Circadian rhythms repeat every 24 hours and almost every living thing has them. They tell animals the best time to hunt, for example, and plants when to flower. Circadian rhythms are influenced by light. When the sun shines through the window in the morning your body clock tells you it's time to wake up. When it's dark your body feels sleepy.

How do they keep you healthy?
Good-quality sleep lets your brain recharge and replace important hormones (chemicals) to keep you healthy. Not listening to your body clock, such as by going to bed late, can mess with your sleep cycle and make you feel tired and irritable the next day. Circadian rhythms also affect energy, digestion and body temperature. In fact, scientists have found that they help our whole body run smoothly. Swathi Yadlapalli is a scientist who studies how people grow and develop. She says, "Almost every cell in the human body has a circadian clock, so there are clocks in most of our organs: the liver, intestines, lungs, skin and more."

Uneven sleep times aren't good for you.

Listen to your body clock
Circadian rhythms are written into people's genes, which are the body's instructions for how to develop and grow. We can't change them but we can listen to what they're telling us. The Sleep Charity, which helps people to sleep better, recommends sticking to regular sleep patterns. So whether you're a night owl who stays up late, or a morning lark who likes to get up early, try going to bed and getting up at the same time every day. It also suggests getting lots of natural light in the morning. Even if the sky is cloudy and grey, this can reset your body clock and make you feel more awake.

Tune into your body clock

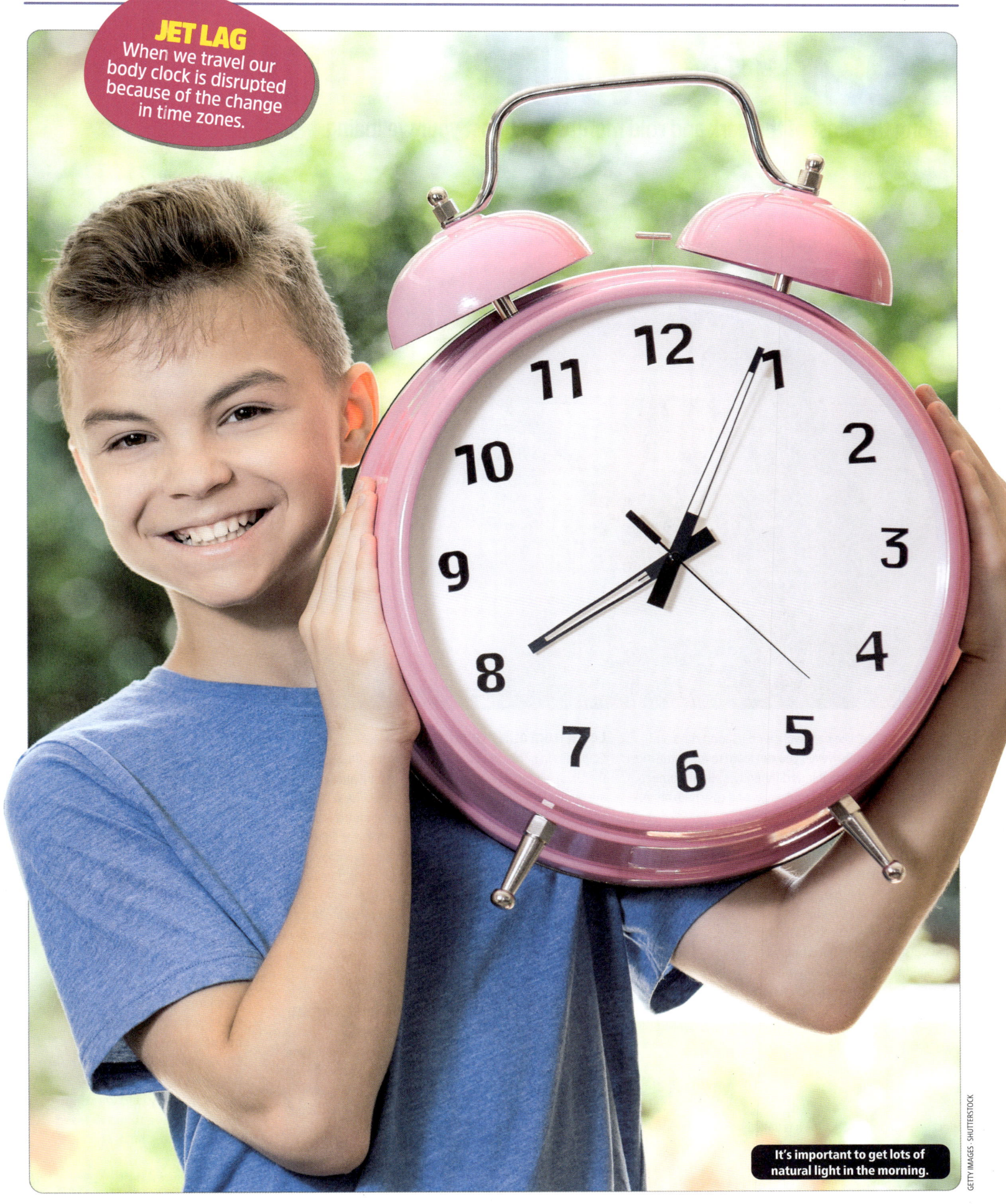

JET LAG
When we travel our body clock is disrupted because of the change in time zones.

It's important to get lots of natural light in the morning.

Physical wellbeing

Beat the winter chills

Making the most of the dark and cold months can boost your wellbeing.

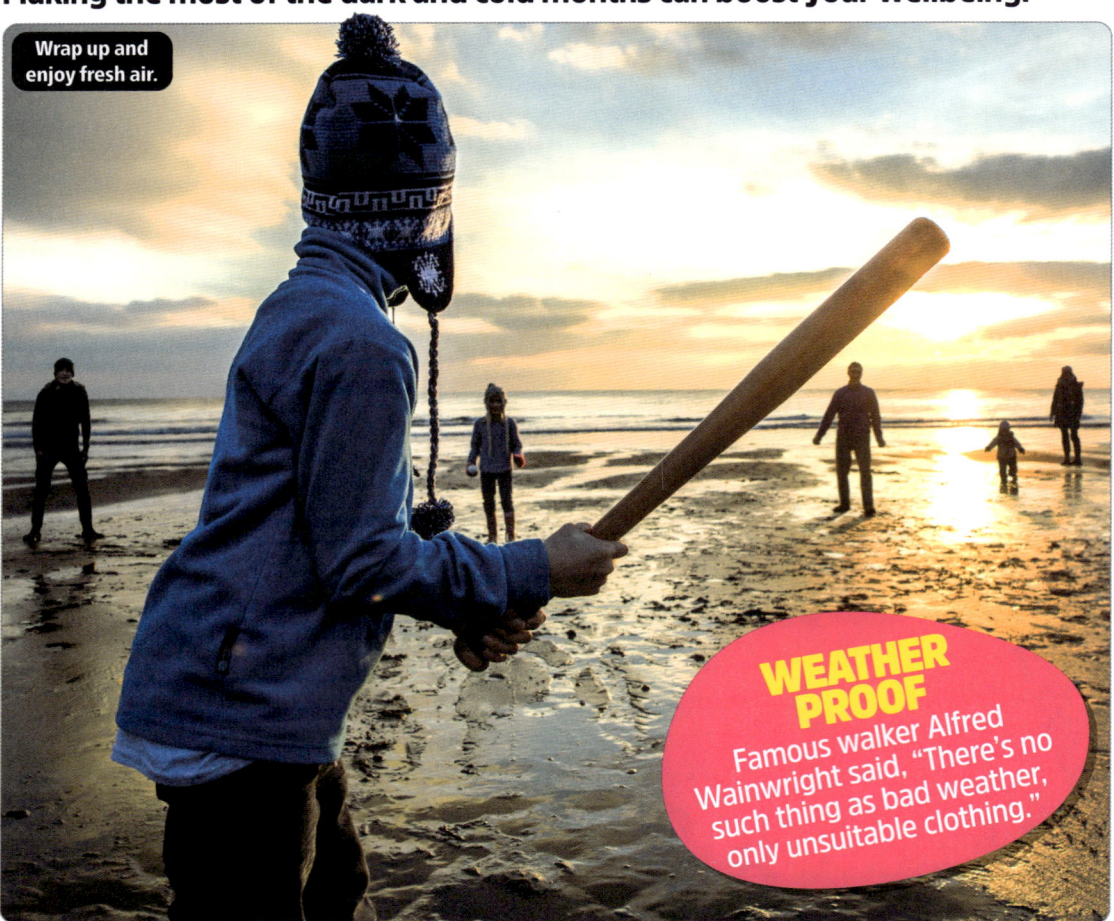

Wrap up and enjoy fresh air.

WEATHER PROOF
Famous walker Alfred Wainwright said, "There's no such thing as bad weather, only unsuitable clothing."

Get outside with friends

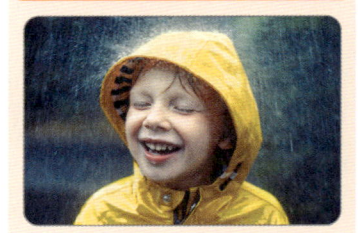

Mental health coach Frances Trussell says it's important for your wellbeing and mental health to keep spending time playing and socialising with friends and family in winter months. "Too much screen time can leave you feeling energetically drained and lead to low moods or just feeling a bit 'meh'. If you've got the right clothes and attitude it can be a blast to play outside in the rain. Studies show that firing up the creative part of your brain improves happiness levels. Painting, baking and crafting can be a great way to have a fun play date."

"I enjoy movie night"

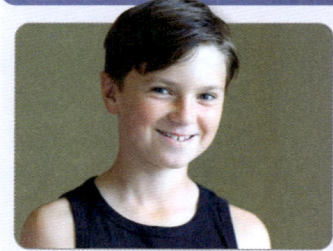

"To get me through the cold and dark winter months I enjoy getting snuggled in my pyjamas and having a movie night with a hot chocolate. I also like playing with the toys that I got for Christmas, and board games with my family. My favourite part about winter is going for walks with my family in really cold weather when you have to get dressed up in big coats, hats, scarves and gloves."
Harrison, aged nine

Winter can feel like hard work with its short days and wet weather. However, you can learn to make the most of the season. By seeing things differently, you can come to love its special mix of brisk, cold walks and cosy relaxation.

Why can the darker months sometimes feel difficult?

During winter there is less daylight and it gets dark earlier. This means you have less time outside to play with friends. It's often rainy, windy and cold, so being outside if you're not wrapped up properly isn't much fun. Frances Trussell, who helps people with their mental health, says, "If you draw a picture of a happy day, it's likely that it would include a bright, sunny sky. So it's no wonder you might find darker winter days more difficult."

Some people have a condition called seasonal affective disorder (SAD), which is linked to a lack of sunlight in winter and vitamin D (your body needs sunlight to make this vitamin). This can make you feel a bit gloomy and grumpy, but there are ways to boost your mood.

Get cosy with family and friends.

Learn from other countries

Countries in northern Europe have even less daylight than the UK in winter. However, Finland, Denmark and Iceland are three of the happiest countries in the world. What helps people in these countries during the dark months is that they don't resist winter or wish it was lighter or warmer. They accept it and they know spring will come. The Danish enjoy "hygge", which is a cosy feeling of being at home with loved ones. They create this comfy setting with candles or fairy lights, and they enjoy delicious food and drink with friends.

Embrace the winter months

You can't change the weather, so make it more enjoyable. Wrap up in waterproof clothing, hats and gloves so you can be snug outside. Get out in the fresh air every day and make the most of any sunshine. Think about how you can feel toasty when you get home, too. Put on a comfy jumper, cuddle a hot water bottle, snuggle under a duvet for a movie night, warm your tummy with soup and drinks – and remember that spring is on its way.

Beat the winter chills

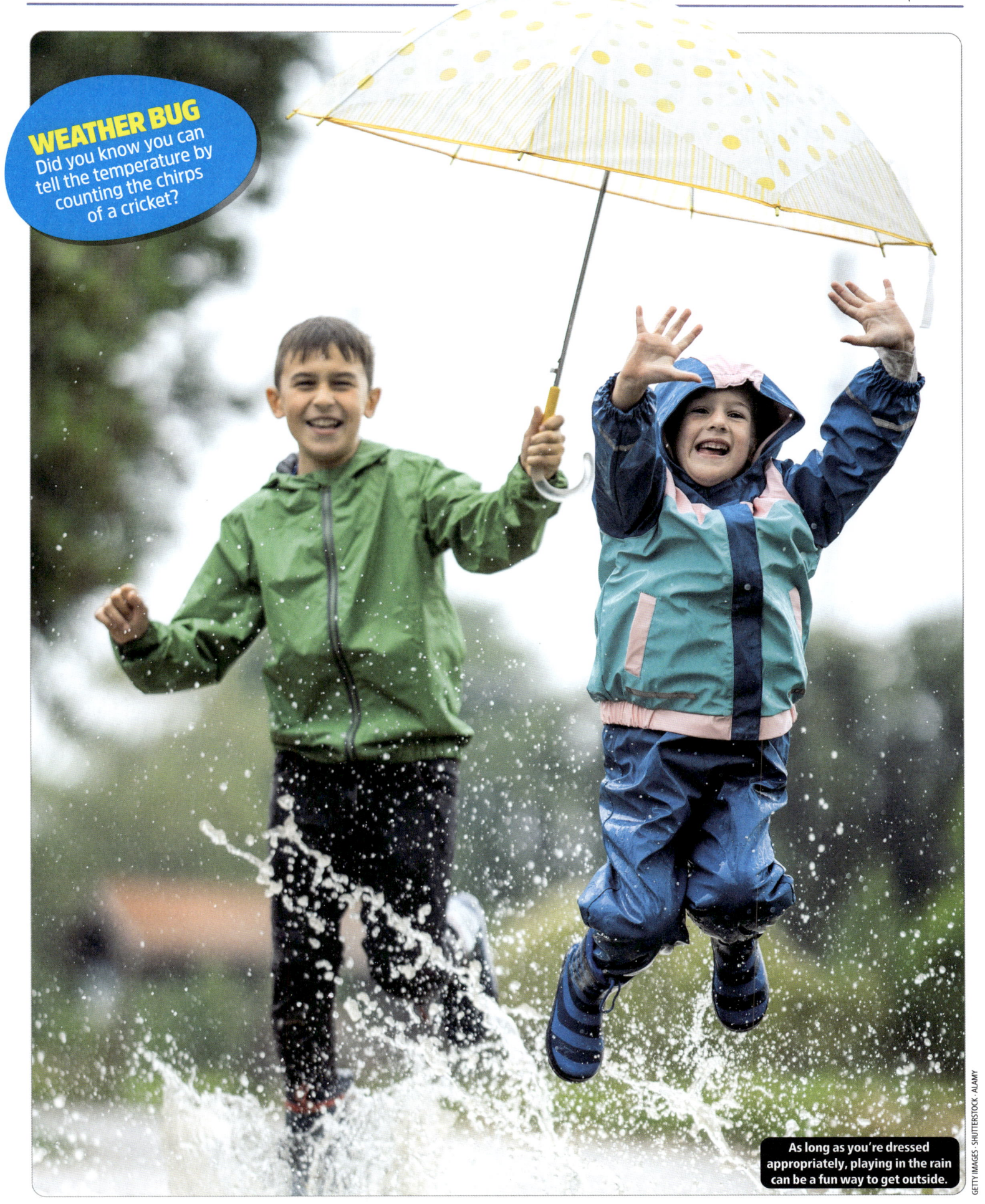

WEATHER BUG
Did you know you can tell the temperature by counting the chirps of a cricket?

As long as you're dressed appropriately, playing in the rain can be a fun way to get outside.

Physical wellbeing

Stay safe in the sun

Enjoy the summer sunshine while staying safe.

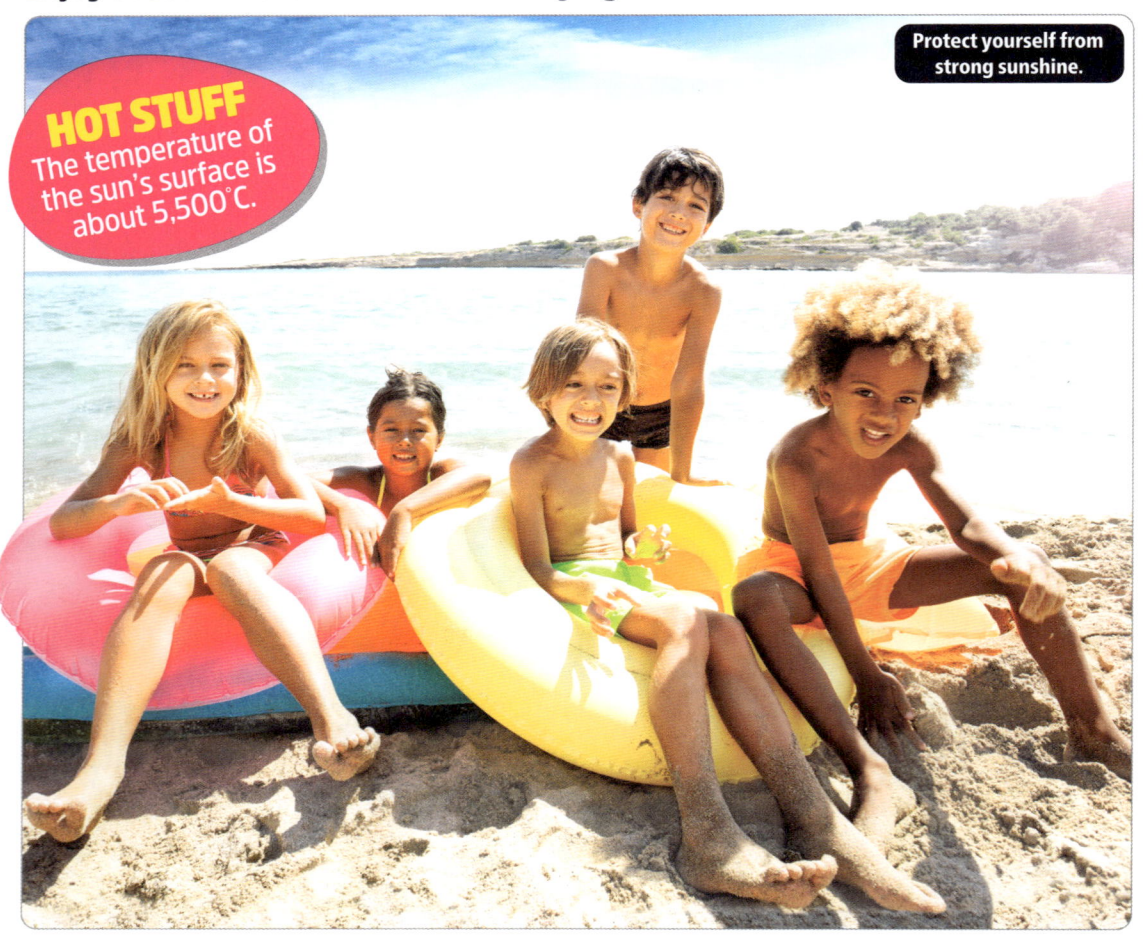

Protect yourself from strong sunshine.

HOT STUFF The temperature of the sun's surface is about 5,500°C.

Summer is the ideal time to be outside having fun in the fresh air and sunshine. It's also very important to protect yourself from the sun's powerful rays.

How the sun affects you
Sunlight boosts your vitamin D levels, which keeps your bones, teeth and muscles healthy. However, from late spring to early autumn the sun's rays are stronger and can damage skin and make you feel unwell. Everyone needs to take care in the sun but the paler your skin the more protection you need. Dr Samantha Anthony, an NHS skin doctor, says, "In strong sunshine the body can heat up quickly, and this can mean you sweat and lose a lot of water. This can make you dehydrated, which can cause headaches, a dry mouth, tiredness, dizziness and fainting."

How to be sun safe
You can have fun in the sun while taking care of yourself by wearing a hat and applying sunscreen with SPF50 (sun protection factor 50). Sweat and swimming washes off sunscreen, so reapply more throughout the day. Wearing sunglasses protects your eyes but it's important to never look directly at the sun. Be sure to drink plenty of water to stay hydrated. The sun is strongest between 11am and 3pm so spend more time indoors or in the shade during this time.

Drink lots of water.

What to do if you're sunburnt
Sunburnt skin is red, hot to touch, can feel sore and itchy, and may blister. If you think you're sunburnt, wash your skin in cold water and apply after-sun cream or aloe vera gel or spray. Don't put ice on it, and try not to scratch peeling skin. Dr Anthony says you should keep your head and body cool. "Move into the shade or indoors and use a cold wet flannel over your skin. Drink cool drinks – sports drinks can help you hydrate. Lie down and rest." It's important to tell an adult straight away if you feel unwell. It's sensible to be careful but playing in the sun is also good for your mood and your health, so head out and have fun.

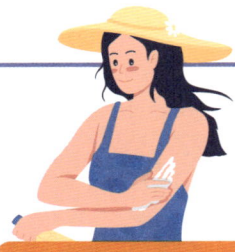

"I try to find shade"

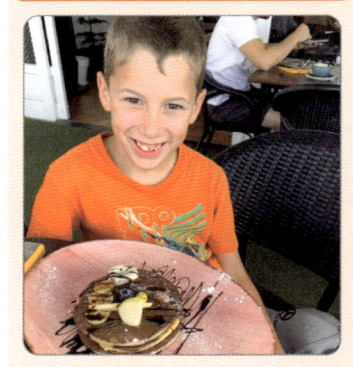

"I love the sunshine (especially if we go on holiday and there's a pool!) but I know it's bad for me to be in the sunshine for too long. When it's really hot and sunny, I drink icy drinks and make sure I don't stay in the sun for too long. I wear light clothes, a baseball cap and sunglasses. I try to find shade to play in, too. If we are at the beach or pool, it's great to jump into the water when it gets too hot!" Zack, aged eight

Remember to slip, slop, slap, seek and slide

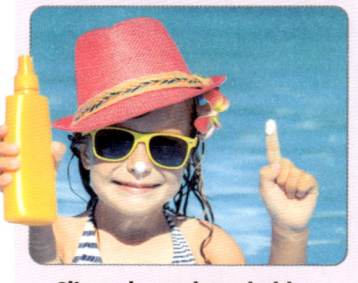

- Slip on loose, breathable clothing to cover your skin.
- Slop on SPF50 sunscreen (don't forget to reapply regularly).
- Slap on a wide-brimmed hat to protect your head and neck.
- Seek shade, especially in the middle of the day.
- Slide on a pair of sunglasses and never look directly at the sun.

Stay safe in the sun

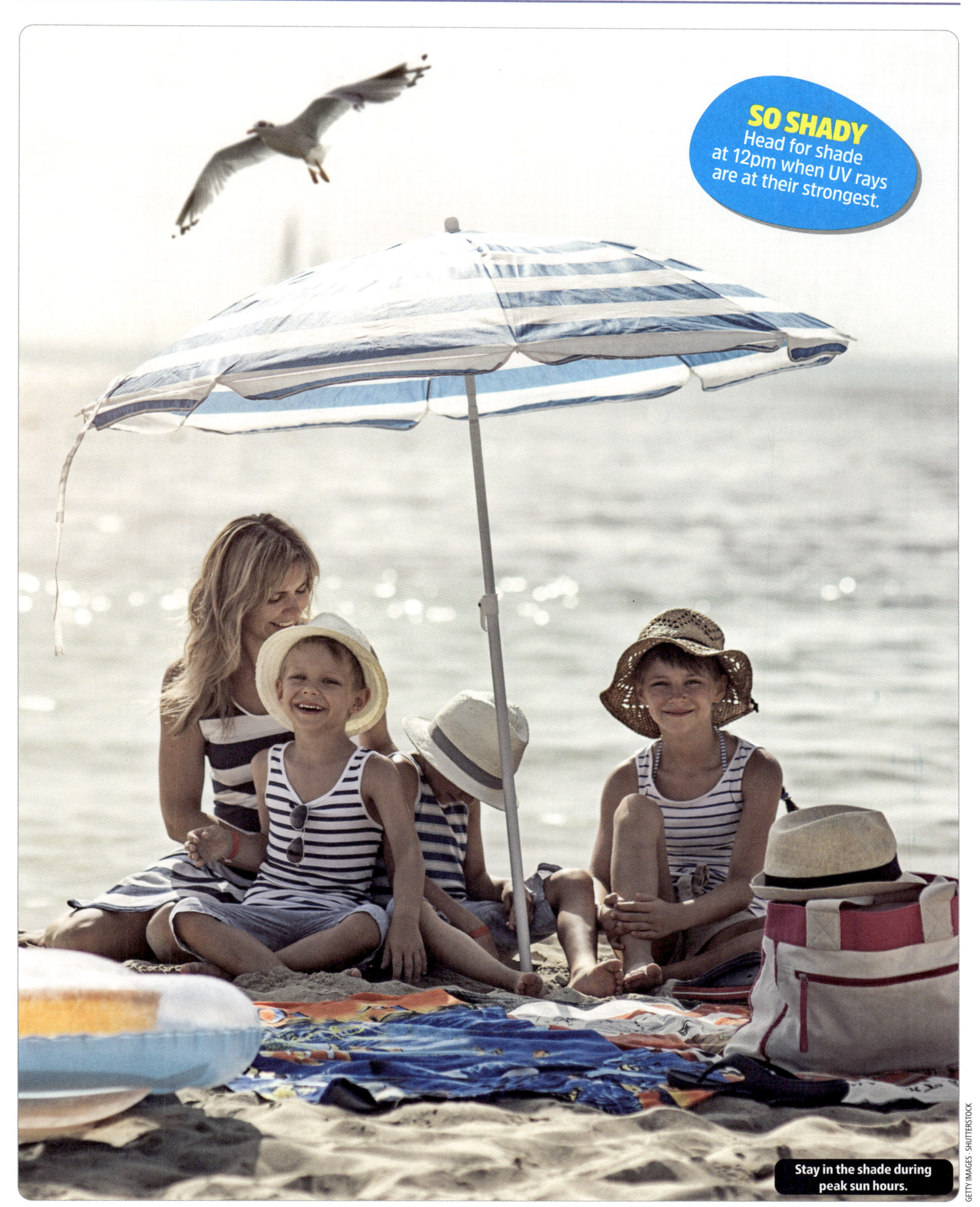

SO SHADY
Head for shade at 12pm when UV rays are at their strongest.

Stay in the shade during peak sun hours.

27

Physical wellbeing

Get to grips with hay fever
Learn to cope with your pollen allergy and make the most of summer.

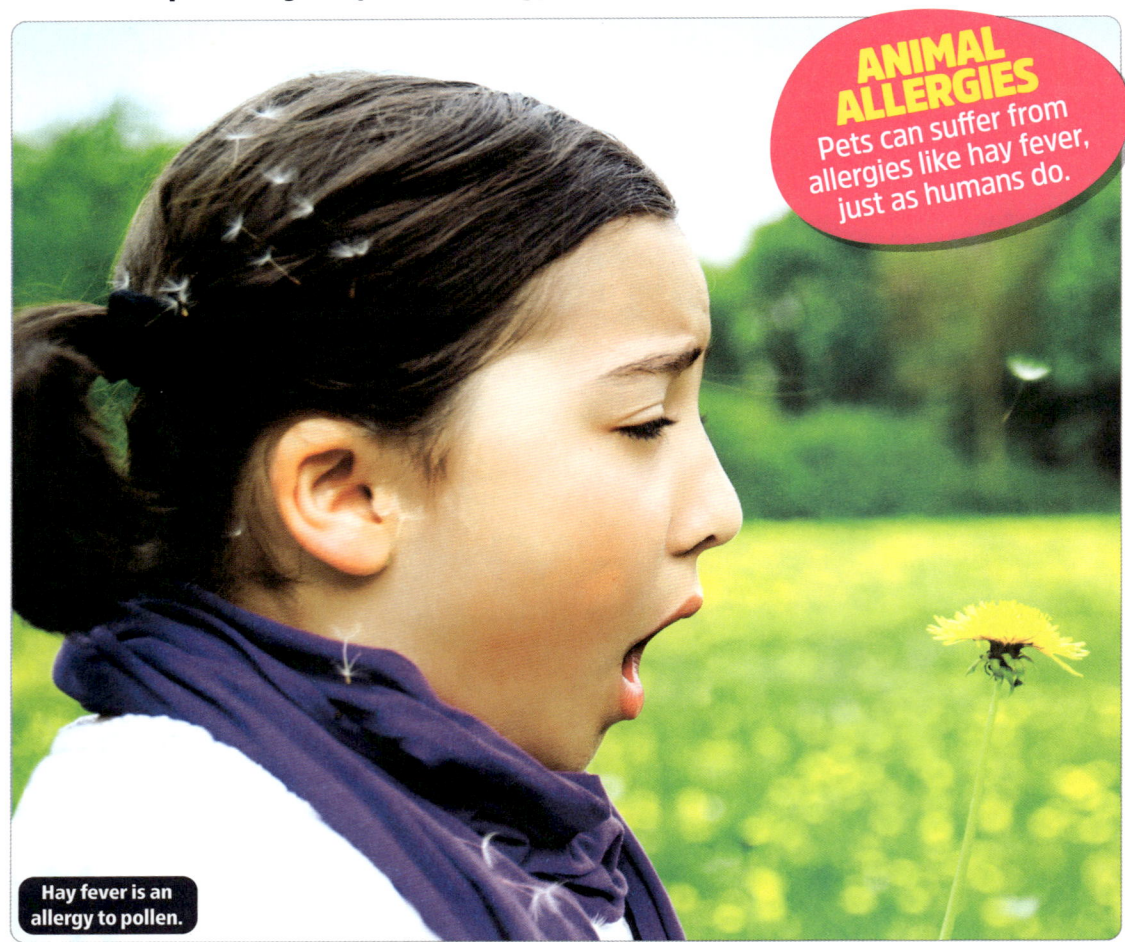

ANIMAL ALLERGIES Pets can suffer from allergies like hay fever, just as humans do.

Hay fever is an allergy to pollen.

Amelie gets hay fever.

Summer means longer days and warmer weather but for many people it also brings itchy eyes and blocked noses. Hay fever affects about 13 million people in the UK. There is no cure but there are ways to manage your symptoms

What is hay fever?
Hay fever is an allergy to pollen – a fine powder that comes from plants. During spring and summer, pollen is released into the air and carried to other plants so they can make seeds. When people breathe in the pollen it can cause an allergic reaction, which might show up as itchy eyes and a runny or blocked nose. These are signs that your body is trying to protect itself from pollen. "Hay fever makes me sneeze a lot and it's irritating when it tickles my nose," says *The Week Junior* reader Amelie, who is 14. It can also disturb your sleep, making you tired.

Why do I get hay fever?
Hay fever is triggered by flower, grass, tree or weed pollen, all of which have different pollen seasons. This is why someone with a tree pollen allergy may get hay fever during the spring, whereas someone who is allergic to grass pollen is more likely to feel bunged up in the summer. Scientists say that allergies are written into our genes, which carry the instructions for how we live and grow.

What can I do about it?
Pollen levels are measured by a pollen count (see panel) and when this is high your symptoms often feel worse.
Dr Runa Ali, an expert in allergies, says, "Wearing glasses or sunglasses can provide some protection for your eyes." She also suggests that sleeping with your window closed can help because pollen levels are higher at night. Medicine like antihistamines can also make you feel better. Always speak to a parent or guardian, and a doctor, and make sure you're supervised before taking any medicine. Also check the dose on the packet. Hay fever symptoms can be annoying but as Ali says, "It's important to remember that typical hay fever symptoms are very mild."

Tips to manage hay fever

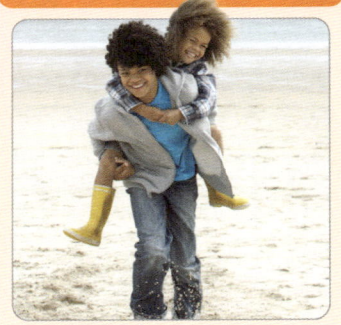

- Try not to walk on grass.
- Stop pollen from going up your nose by putting petroleum jelly around and inside your nostrils.
- Have a shower or change your clothes after you have been outside.
- If you can, escape to the beach where pollen levels are usually low.

What is the pollen count?

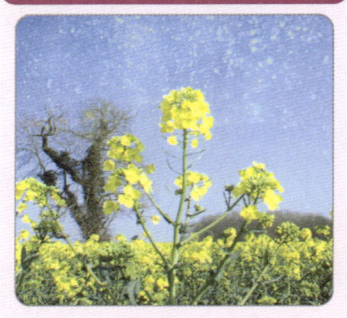

The pollen count is the average amount of pollen grains found within a cubic metre (a cube that measures one metre on each side) of air over 24 hours. The grains are collected using a Burkard trap. This draws air in and catches pollen grains on sticky paper. These are counted using a microscope. A count of 50 or above is high and usually causes hay fever symptoms. The Met Office has a five-day pollen forecast on its website.

28

Get to grips with hay fever

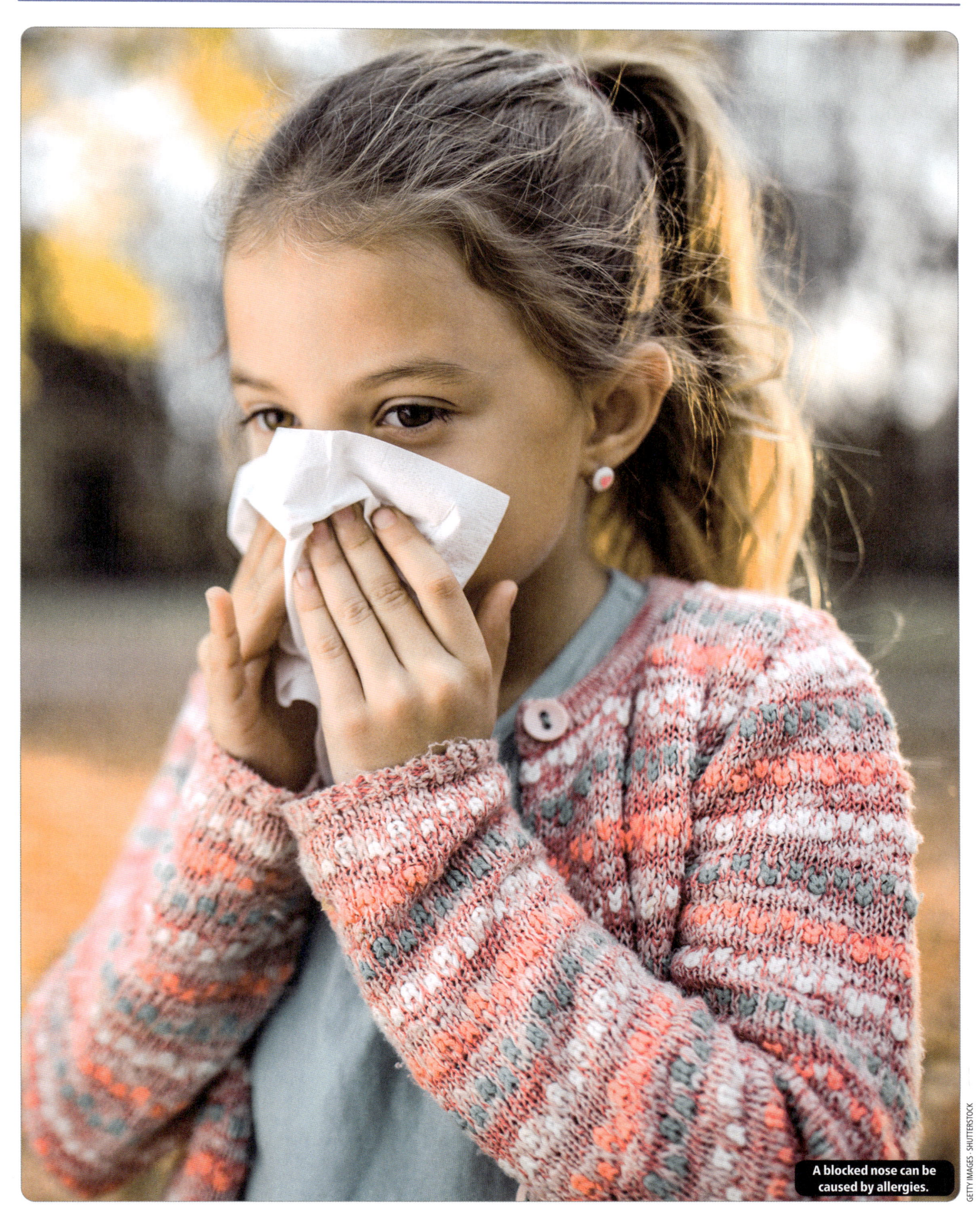

A blocked nose can be caused by allergies.

Physical wellbeing

Speak up for a better internet
Have your say about how life online can be improved for our safety.

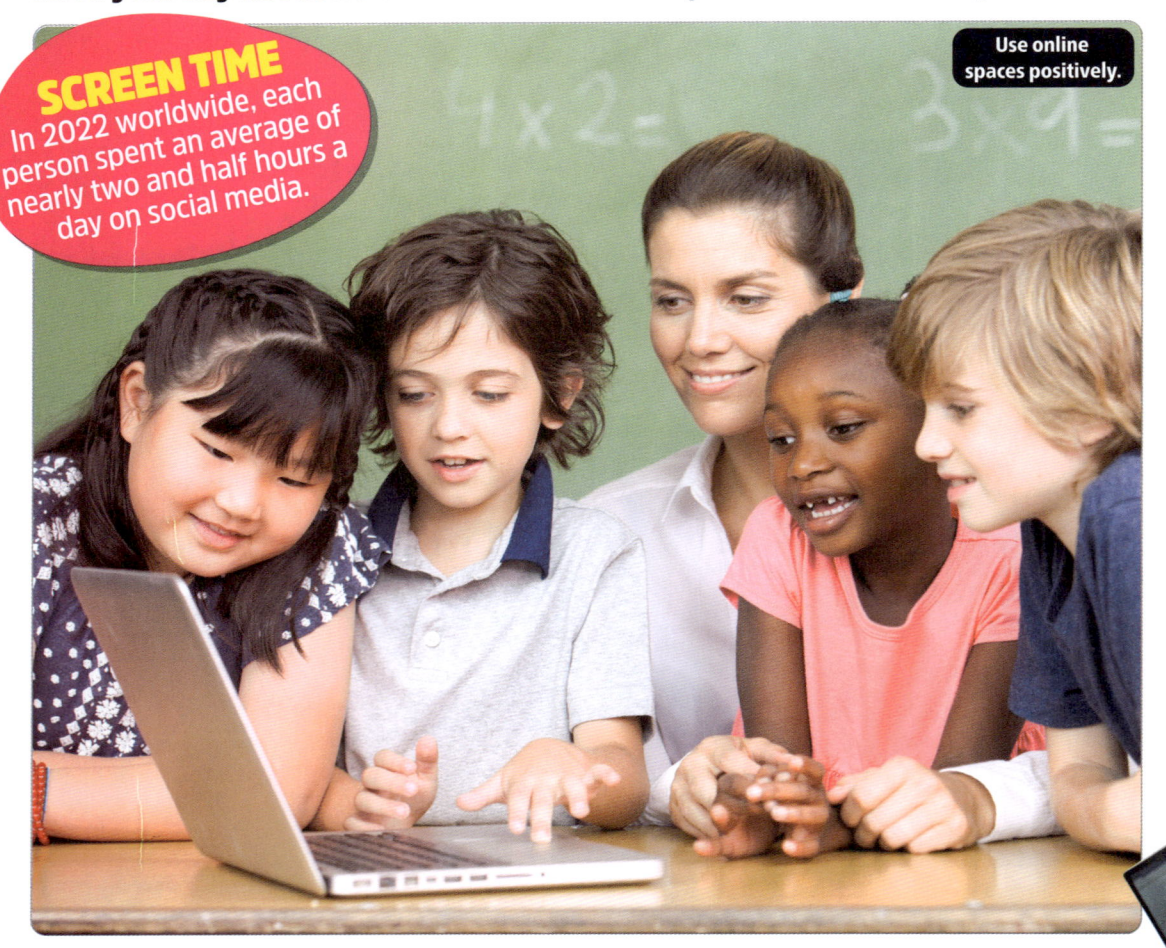

SCREEN TIME
In 2022 worldwide, each person spent an average of nearly two and half hours a day on social media.

Use online spaces positively.

Tips for digital self-care
Gwen Taylor from Glitch shares tips to look after yourself online.

- Check your privacy settings on social media – can everyone see your accounts or send you a message? Make sure only people you trust can talk to you online.
- If someone is being abusive, don't talk to them. Block them and talk to a trusted adult about what happened.
- Unfollow accounts that aren't making you happy.
- If being online isn't making you feel good, take a break. Uninstall apps or log out.

Online or offline?

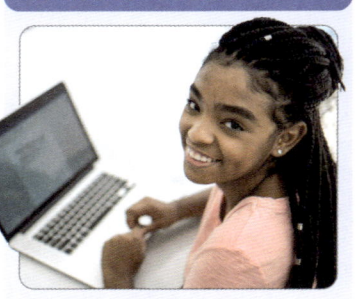

Use this table to have a discussion with friends or family about the benefits and drawbacks of the internet.

In real life there are accepted rules that everybody follows. For example, you shouldn't eat with your mouth open; in the UK people drive on the left; and the only place to join a queue is at the back. Online, the rules aren't as clear and it can be hard to know how to behave.

What is being safe online?
You probably know the basics of being safe online: don't give personal details to somebody you don't know, and check trusted sites to spot a fake story. Gwen Taylor is from the charity Glitch, which works to end online abuse. She says, "It's also about whether you're able to do the things you love without feeling worried or upset." This is important so everybody can join in. Glitch's research found that 43% of girls don't share their opinions online in case they are criticised.

Talk to an adult if someone has been unkind.

What should I do if I experience online abuse?
Cyberbullying – bullying that takes place online – is never ok. The first thing to do is to tell a trusted adult about what's happening. If another person has been unkind, or they post content that frightens you, you can report it to the social media or gaming platform where it happened. Taylor advises taking a screenshot of the abuse before deleting it because this will help you to report it and help others to help you. Even though it can be tempting to say something unkind in return, this can make things worse, so try to stay calm. You can also call Childline on 0800 1111 or visit childline.org.uk

Being a good digital citizen
How you act online is just as important as how others treat you. "Good digital citizens use online spaces positively, which means treating everybody online with kindness and respect," says Taylor. If you've shared something you shouldn't have, or left someone out of an online group, it's never too late to say sorry and fix the situation (such as taking the post down or adding the person to your group). If you notice somebody is being cyberbullied, consider reporting it and getting in touch with the person being treated badly to make sure they're ok.

	Better offline	Better online	Unsure
Talking to friends	☐	☐	☐
Playing games	☐	☐	☐
Learning	☐	☐	☐
Seeking help	☐	☐	☐
Shopping	☐	☐	☐

Speak up for a better internet

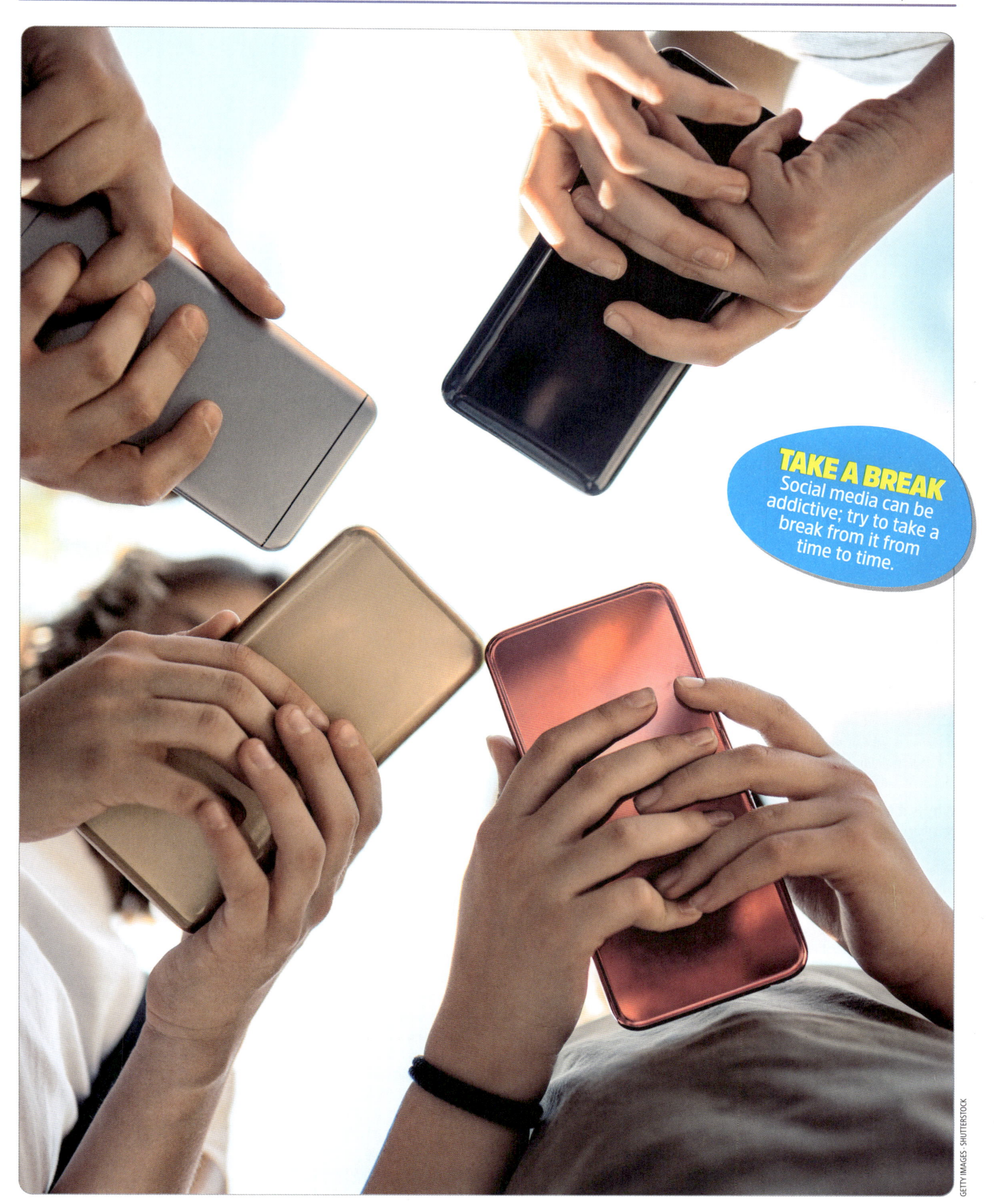

TAKE A BREAK
Social media can be addictive; try to take a break from it from time to time.

31

Physical wellbeing

Make money your friend
Keeping your cash safe and secure can make you feel more confident.

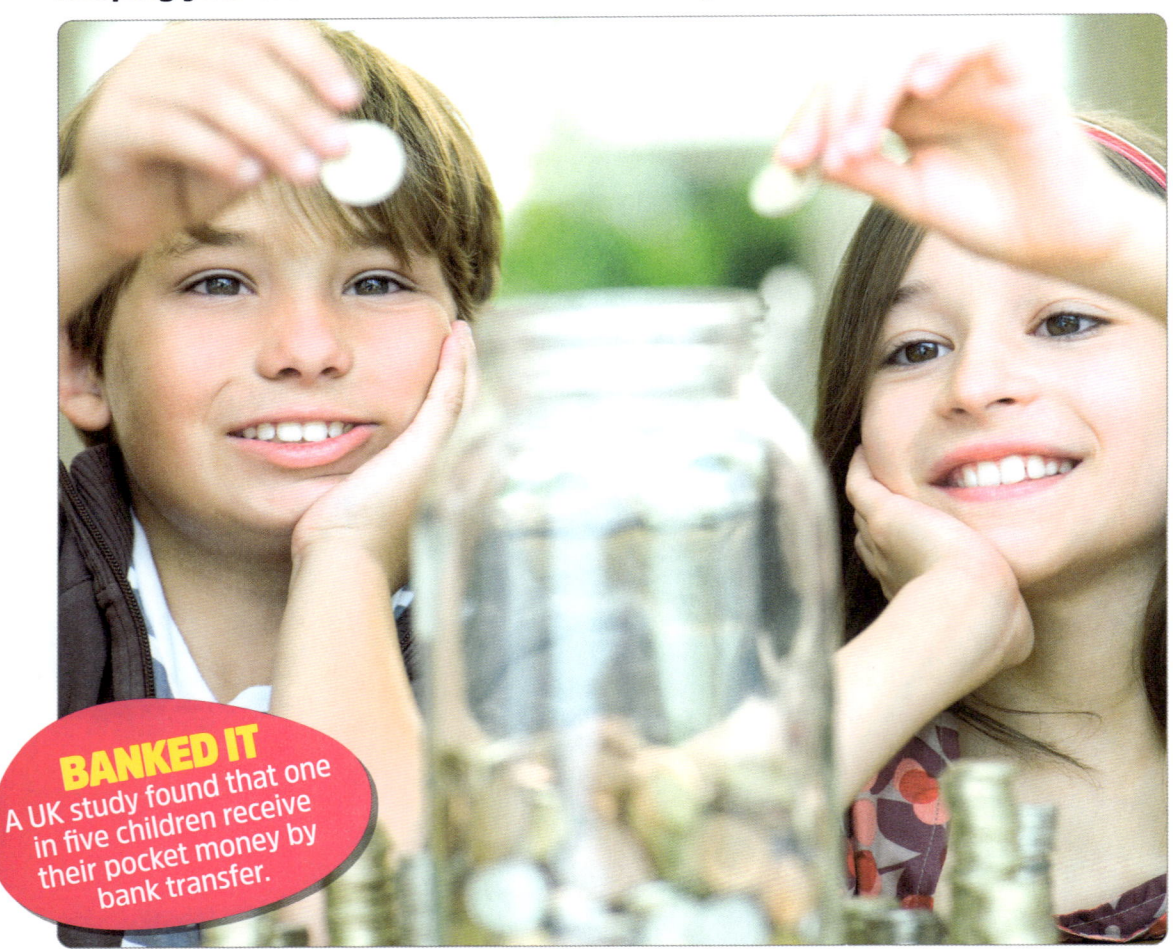

BANKED IT
A UK study found that one in five children receive their pocket money by bank transfer.

However you feel about money, it plays a big role in life. Understanding how it works can make you feel more confident and happy and can help you reach your goals.

Why is it helpful to understand money?
Whether you want to make a million pounds or are comfortable with just enough, understanding money is an important skill to have. Kalpana Fitzpatrick is a money expert and author of *Get to Know: Money*. She tells *The Week Junior* that understanding money isn't just about maths and numbers. "It's a tool to help you live a better life the way you want it," she says. So if you dream of buying a new guitar or travelling around the world one day, knowing when to spend and save your cash will help you.

How can you manage money better?
Fitzpatrick suggests treating money the same way you would a good friend. "You need to communicate, understand boundaries and be able to ask for help if you need it," she explains. So if you need a certain amount of money to buy a computer game, for example, look after the money you already have. This could mean keeping it safe in a savings account so that it builds up, or not spending it on things you don't need. As well as helping you reach your goals, this will help you build a happy, healthy relationship with money in the future.

Sell cakes or drinks to earn cash.

Where can you learn more?
"Don't be afraid to ask questions and get advice," says Fitzpatrick. Try talking to parents, carers and teachers, or find reliable news sources like books and BBC Bitesize. "It's helpful to be nosy," she says. According to a study by GoHenry, the debit card and financial education app, more than 70% of young people in the UK say earning their own money is important, and many are doing this by starting their own businesses. Think up some money-making ideas, such as making and selling cakes or jewellery, and learn while you earn. "Being good with money isn't about being rich or comparing yourself to others," says Fitzpatrick. "It's about knowing what matters to you."

Go treasure hunting

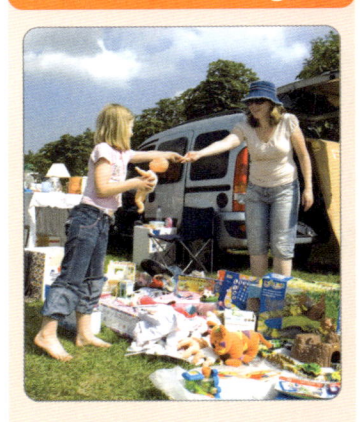

"Collectibles" are anything that might be valuable to a collector. Even though they don't always look special, they can be worth a lot, like the page of a Spider-Man comic that sold for £2.7 million in 2022. You could search charity shops and car boot sales for football cards or old toys that people might start collecting one day. You never know, the treasures you find might go up in value in the future.

How to manage money

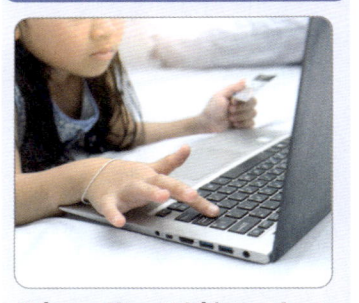

Kalpana Fitzpatrick's top tips to help look after your money:

- **Set a goal.** If you really want something but don't have enough money to buy it, make a plan to save up.
- **Before spending, work out if you're buying something you want** (for example sweets) or something you need, like pens for school. Ask yourself if it's worth it.
- **Instead of stuffing your savings into a money box, open a savings account** (with help from an adult) and watch your money grow.

Make money your friend

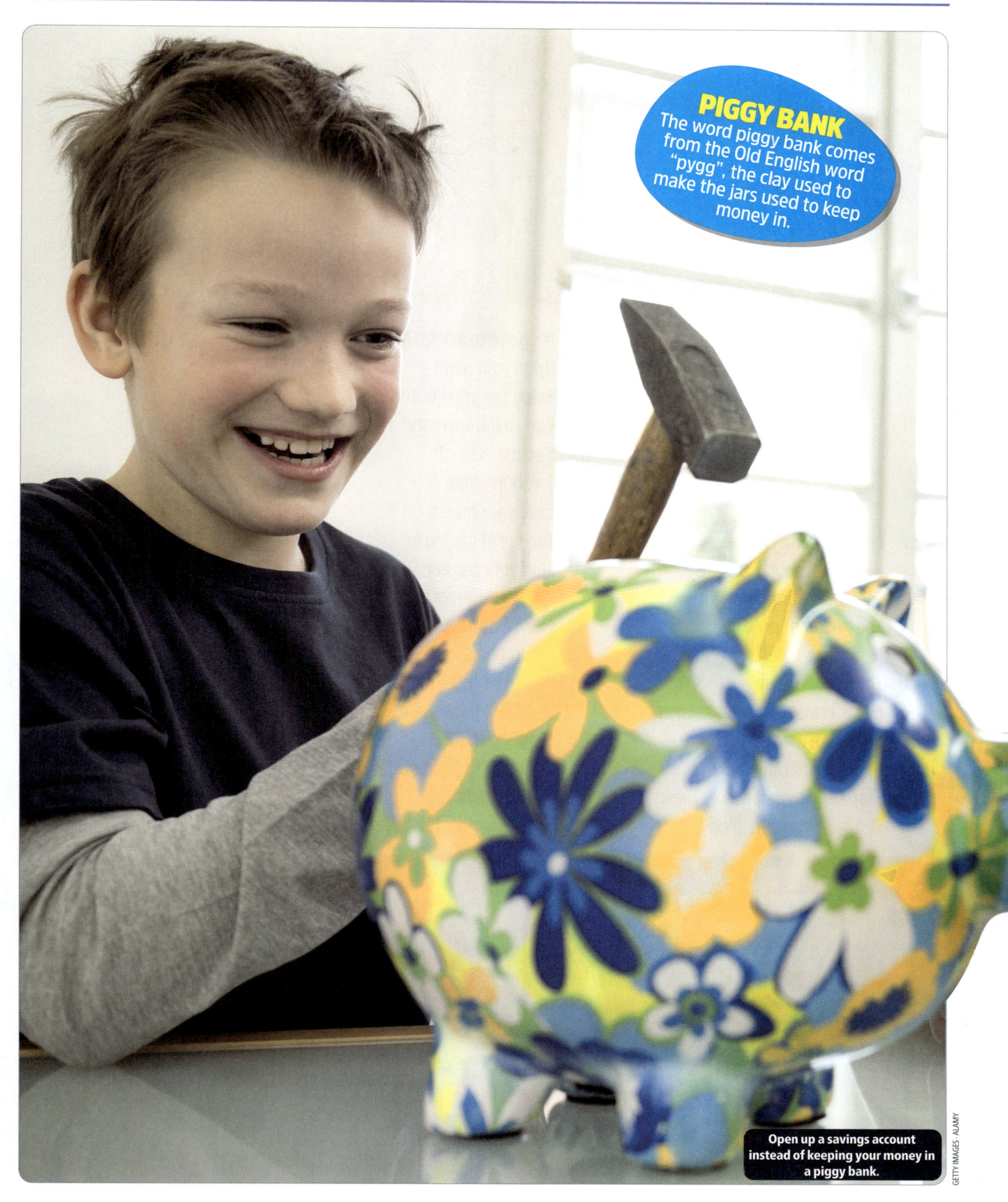

PIGGY BANK
The word piggy bank comes from the Old English word "pygg", the clay used to make the jars used to keep money in.

Open up a savings account instead of keeping your money in a piggy bank.

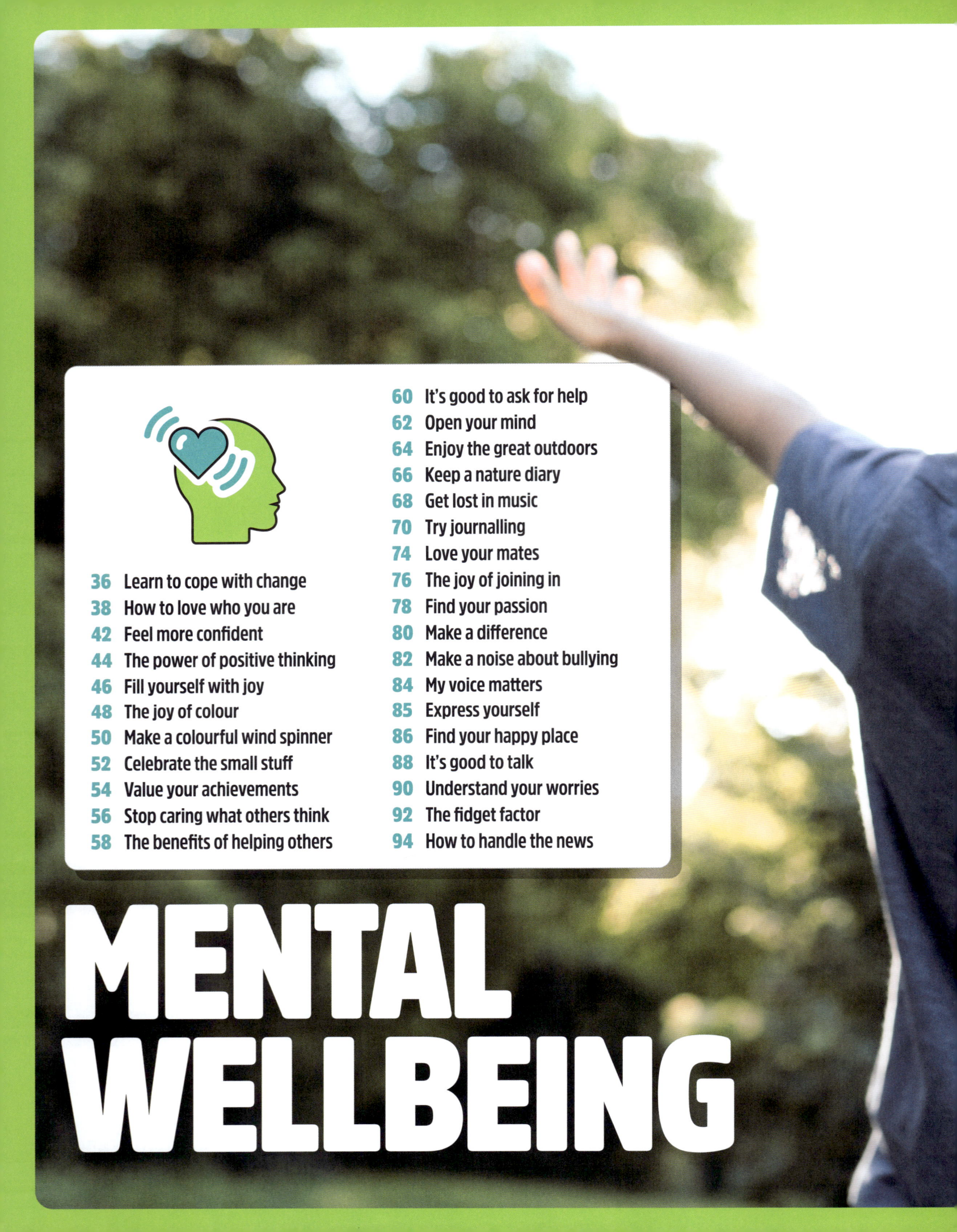

36	Learn to cope with change
38	How to love who you are
42	Feel more confident
44	The power of positive thinking
46	Fill yourself with joy
48	The joy of colour
50	Make a colourful wind spinner
52	Celebrate the small stuff
54	Value your achievements
56	Stop caring what others think
58	The benefits of helping others
60	It's good to ask for help
62	Open your mind
64	Enjoy the great outdoors
66	Keep a nature diary
68	Get lost in music
70	Try journalling
74	Love your mates
76	The joy of joining in
78	Find your passion
80	Make a difference
82	Make a noise about bullying
84	My voice matters
85	Express yourself
86	Find your happy place
88	It's good to talk
90	Understand your worries
92	The fidget factor
94	How to handle the news

MENTAL WELLBEING

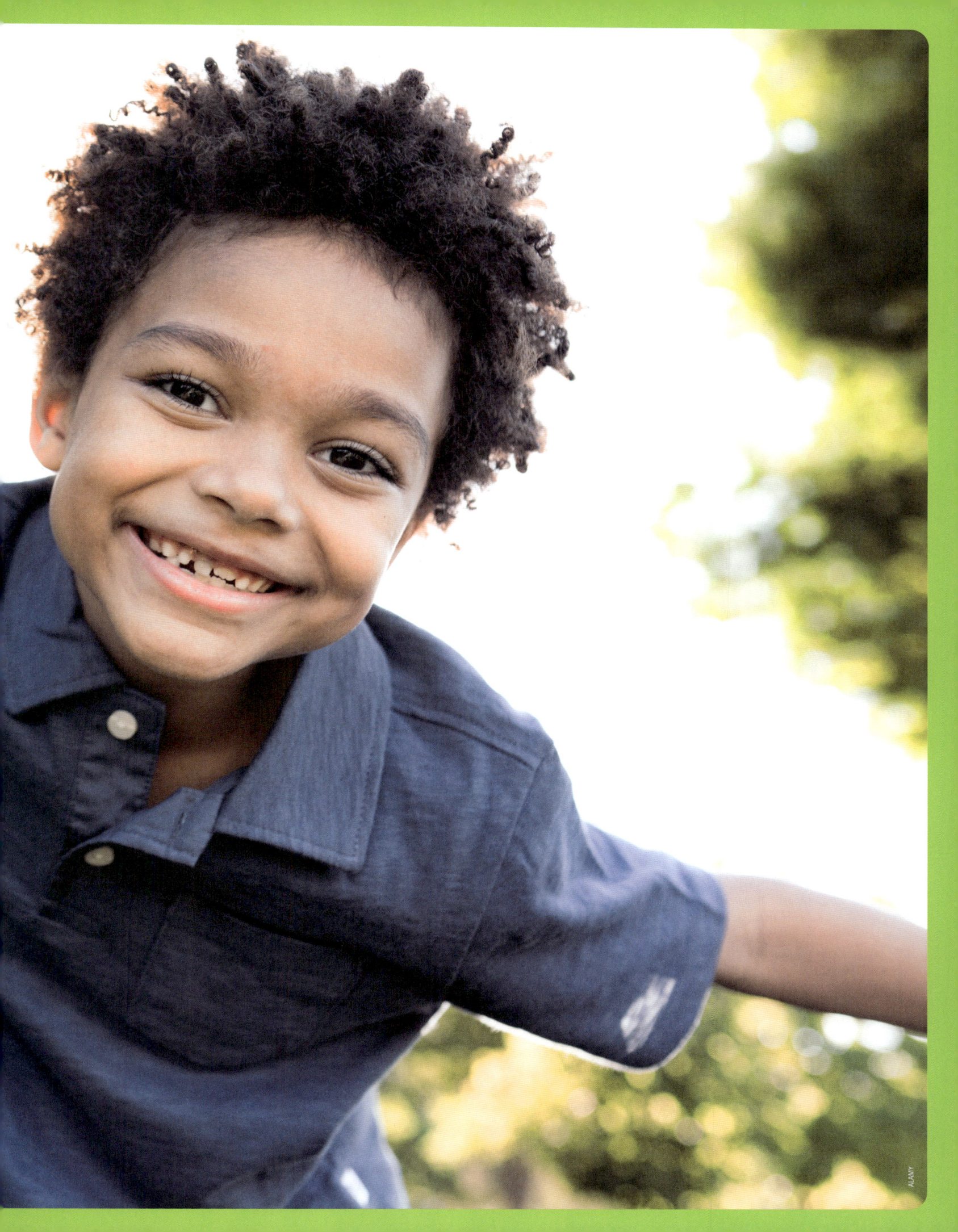

Mental wellbeing

Learn to cope with change

Learning to cope with change will help you look forward to new experiences.

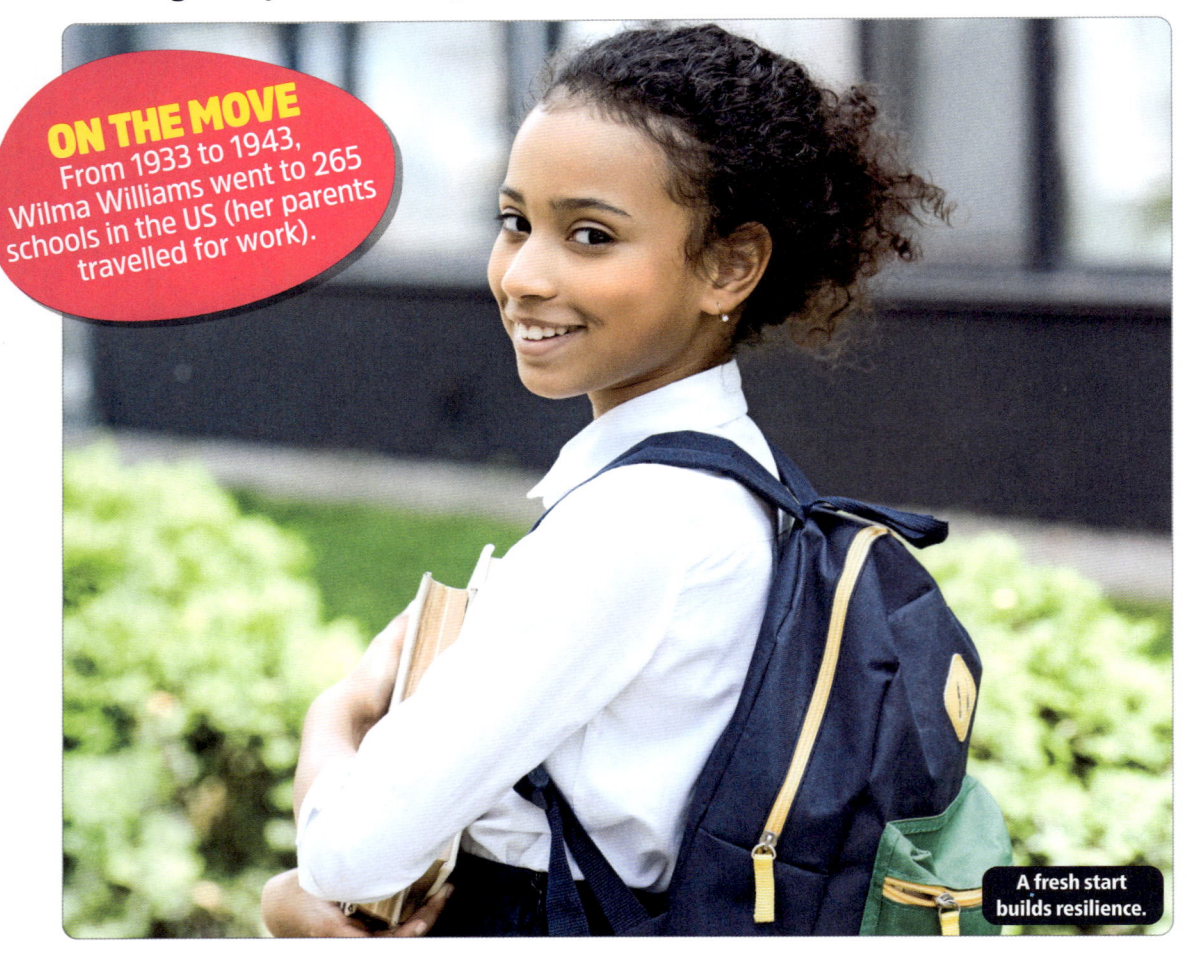

ON THE MOVE
From 1933 to 1943, Wilma Williams went to 265 schools in the US (her parents travelled for work).

A fresh start builds resilience.

Top tips for managing change well

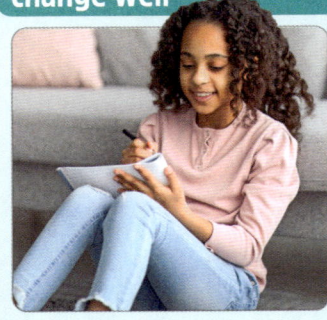

- Take one day at a time. Focus on the day ahead instead of worrying about what might happen further in the future.
- Think about changes you've been through before, like joining a new sports team or after-school club, and how you coped then.
- Celebrate endings and remember the good times, for example by talking about or writing down memories of your old class or school.

Starting secondary school

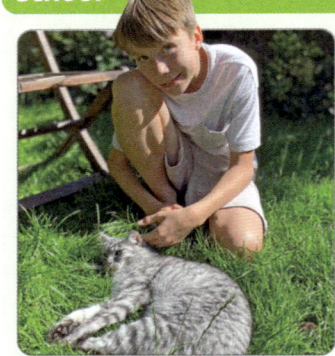

"I am excited about meeting new kids and teachers, but I am also nervous that some subjects might be hard and it will take a while to make new friends. In the holidays I met up with someone who will be in my form and that has helped me relax, and I will still keep in touch with my old friends who are going to different schools."
Ben, aged 11

Are you starting a new school or class this year? This is something that everyone goes through and it can teach you skills that will help you deal with change in the future.

Change happens
Change is a normal part of life. It might be leaving your old school and starting a new one, joining a different class or moving to a new home, and it can feel strange and scary. Dr Aaron Balick is an author and expert in thoughts and feelings. He says that although you can't prepare for every change that's going to happen, you can learn how to deal with it. "Getting skilled up in dealing with change will help you for the rest of your life," Balick says.

Make the most of change
Even if you're excited about starting a new school, you can still feel anxious, sad or worried. Rebecca Wilkinson-Quinn from Place2Be, a charity that supports schools, says these are "normal feelings to have", especially if you're leaving friends or favourite teachers behind. Try to talk about these feelings to family or friends. Balick says that if you're sad it's a sign you've had a good experience that you're sorry to leave behind. If you're not sad then you are probably ready for a new start that will challenge you.

It's ok to feel worried.

Making change easier to manage
Wilkinson-Quinn recommends expressing your feelings in a way that feels good to you. "This may be through talking, art, music or something else," she says. Trying to see both sides of the change can also be helpful. "List the things that are different, but also the things that are the same," explains Wilkinson-Quinn. "Think about the positives that have come from the change – it may surprise you."
Balick says that change is a chance to become more resilient and learn to deal with life's challenges. Think of school as a good exercise. "Try to stay aware of your feelings as they develop over the first few weeks, and then compare them to what you had expected – you'll be surprised," he explains. "Next time big change comes, you'll know how to face it even better."

Learn to cope with change

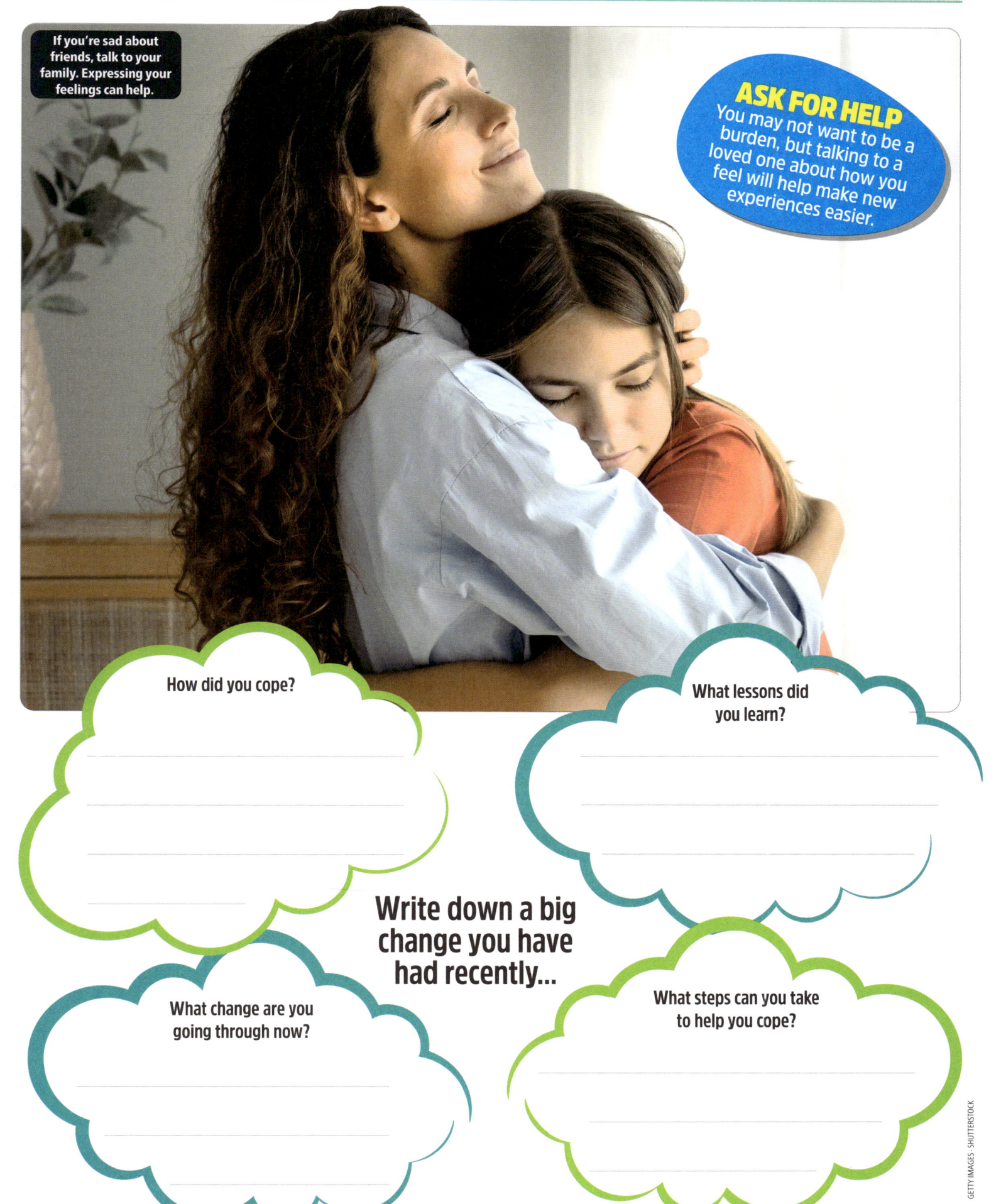

If you're sad about friends, talk to your family. Expressing your feelings can help.

ASK FOR HELP
You may not want to be a burden, but talking to a loved one about how you feel will help make new experiences easier.

Write down a big change you have had recently...

How did you cope?

What lessons did you learn?

What change are you going through now?

What steps can you take to help you cope?

Mental wellbeing

How to love who you are
Learning to love yourself helps you overcome challenges.

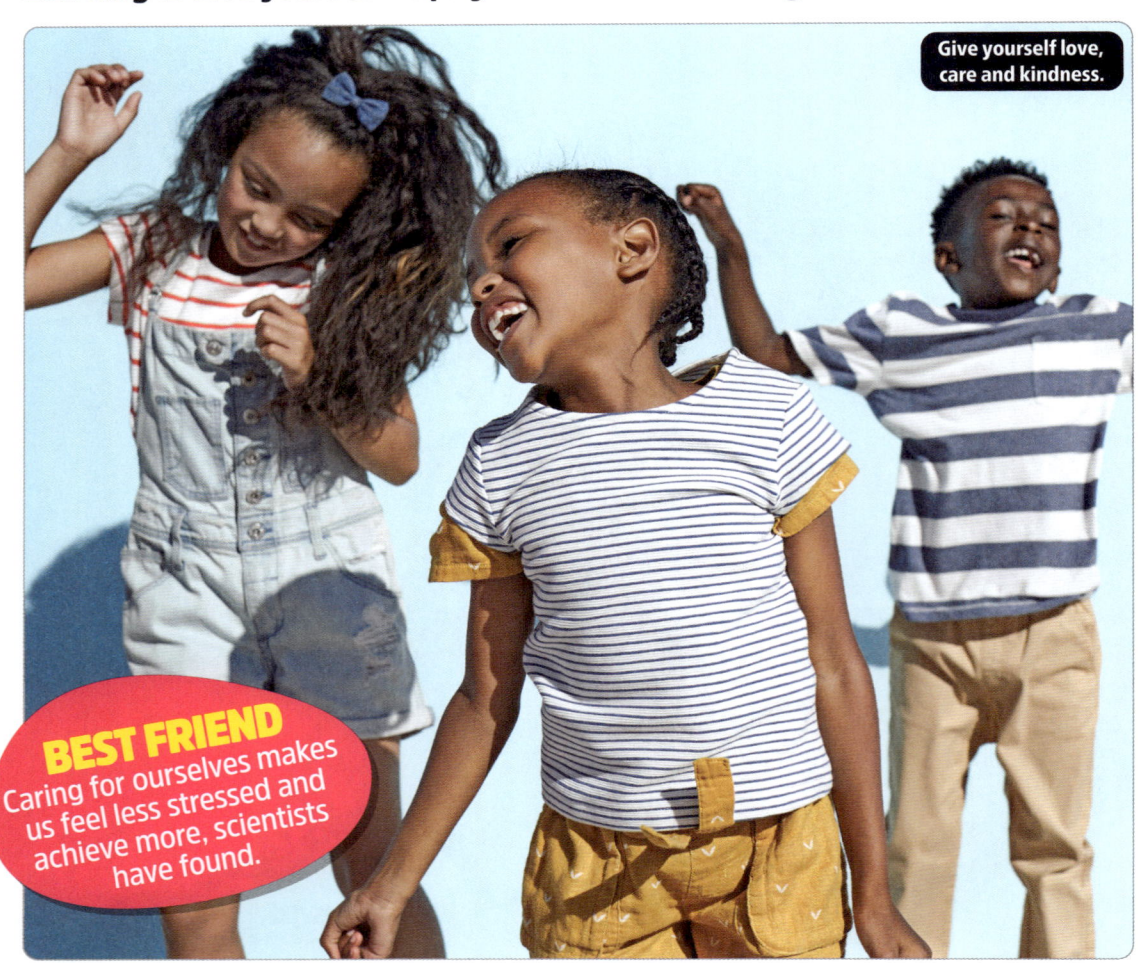

Give yourself love, care and kindness.

BEST FRIEND Caring for ourselves makes us feel less stressed and achieve more, scientists have found.

Why not find a new friend this year – yourself! Being treated with kindness, respect and love are things you would expect from a good friendship and you shouldn't have to go far to find them. Start by being your own friend.

What does self-love mean?
Loving yourself, also called self-love, means being as kind to yourself as you are to others. Imagine your best friend is worried or upset, then think about how you'd support them and try to make them feel better. Self-love means giving yourself the love, care and respect you might give your friends and family. Becky Goddard-Hill, the author of *Create Your Own Confidence*, tells *The Week Junior* it means valuing yourself at all times. "It's speaking to yourself with kindness and encouragement, and it means taking really good care of your body and mind."

Why does it matter?
Learning to love who you are strengthens your self-esteem (how you feel about yourself). The mental health charity YoungMinds says this makes you believe in yourself and feel that you deserve good things – such as kind friends and fun experiences. It doesn't mean you'll be happy all the time, YoungMinds explains, but when you do face challenges they'll be easier to overcome. Studies show that self-love can help friendships, schoolwork and health. "There is always someone looking out for you," says Goddard-Hill, "because that person is you."

Write down your strengths.

Love yourself better
Start by being kind, especially if you make a mistake. Instead of being angry, tell yourself that everyone gets things wrong sometimes. Then work out what you could do differently next time. Try not to compare yourself to others and remember that no-one is perfect. Focus on yourself instead. Goddard-Hill recommends writing down your strengths and asking your family and friends for their thoughts. "Keep the list somewhere safe and look at it often to remind yourself you are amazing," she says. Before you go to bed, think about three things that went well for you that day. "This will help you see the positives in your life," says Goddard-Hill.

Positive self-talk

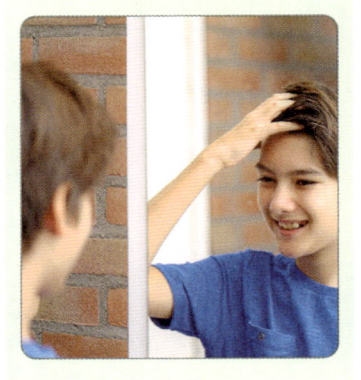

An "affirmation" is saying a positive statement to yourself. Becky Goddard-Hill recommends doing this three times every morning to give yourself a boost. Here are some ideas, can you think of any more?

- I like who I am.
- I can do this.
- I am a good friend.

Take time out for you

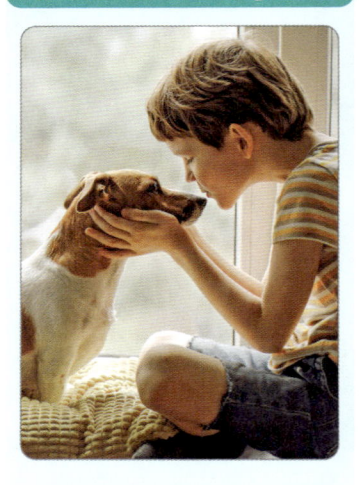

Spend 15 minutes a day giving yourself the attention you deserve, starting with:

- Listening to your favourite music.
- Going for a walk or bike ride.
- Cuddling your pet.
- Reading a book in bed.
- Enjoying a mug of hot chocolate.

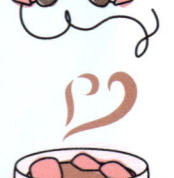

38

How to love who you are

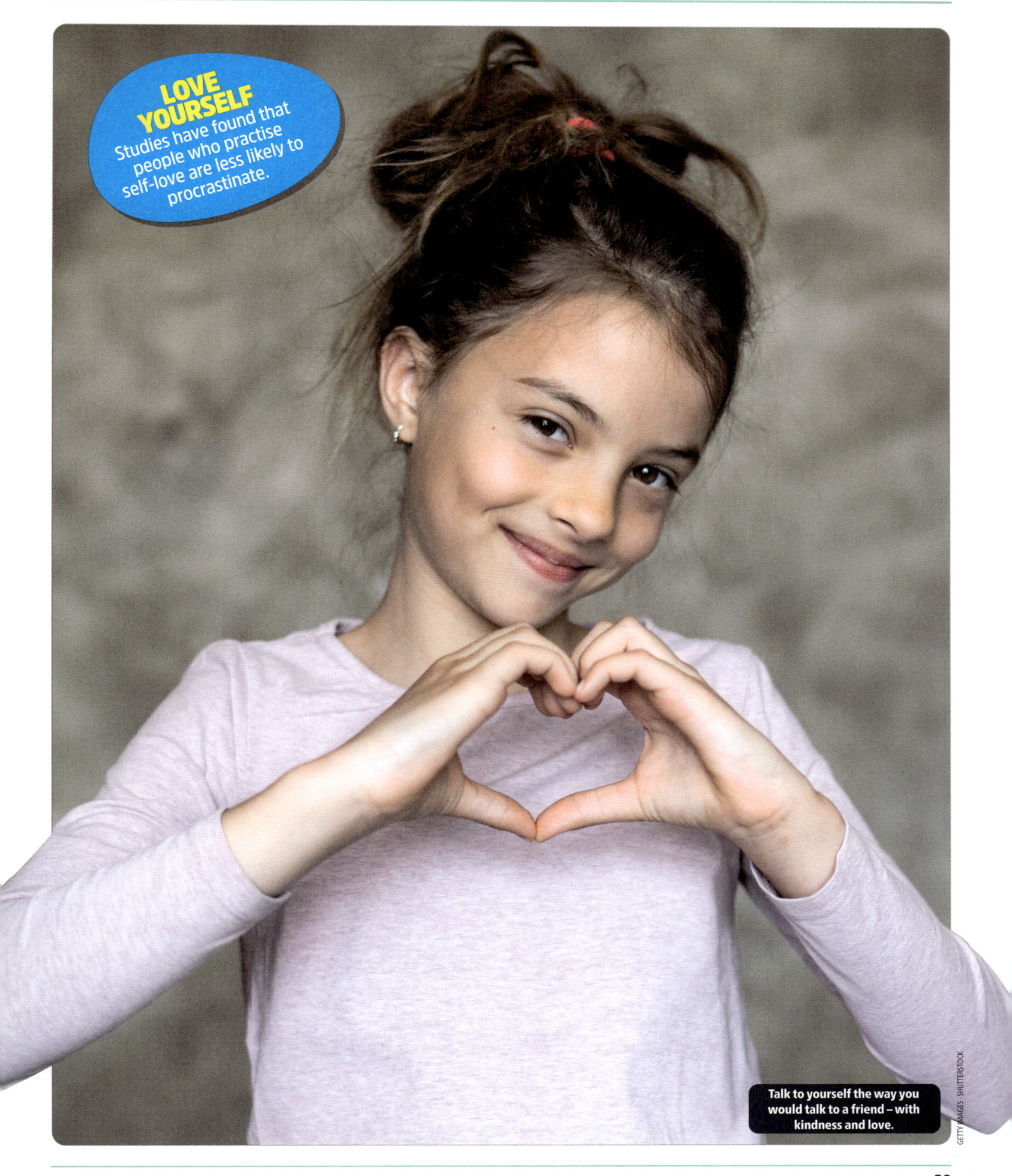

LOVE YOURSELF
Studies have found that people who practise self-love are less likely to procrastinate.

Talk to yourself the way you would talk to a friend – with kindness and love.

Mental wellbeing

THINGS I LOVE ABOUT ME...

Draw a self-portrait of yourself, then fill in the hearts with things you love about yourself:

How to love who you are

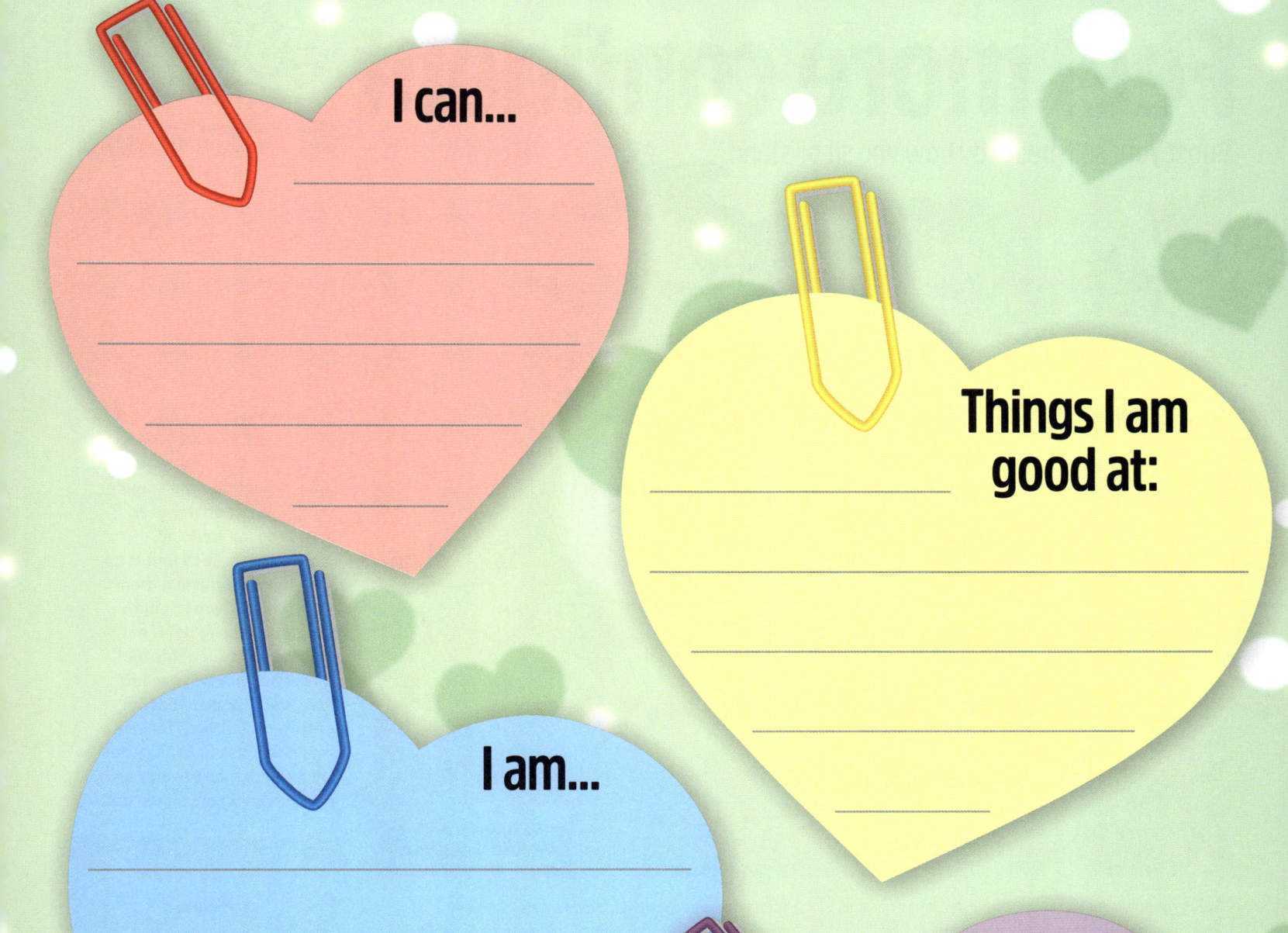

I can...

Things I am good at:

I am...

I love...

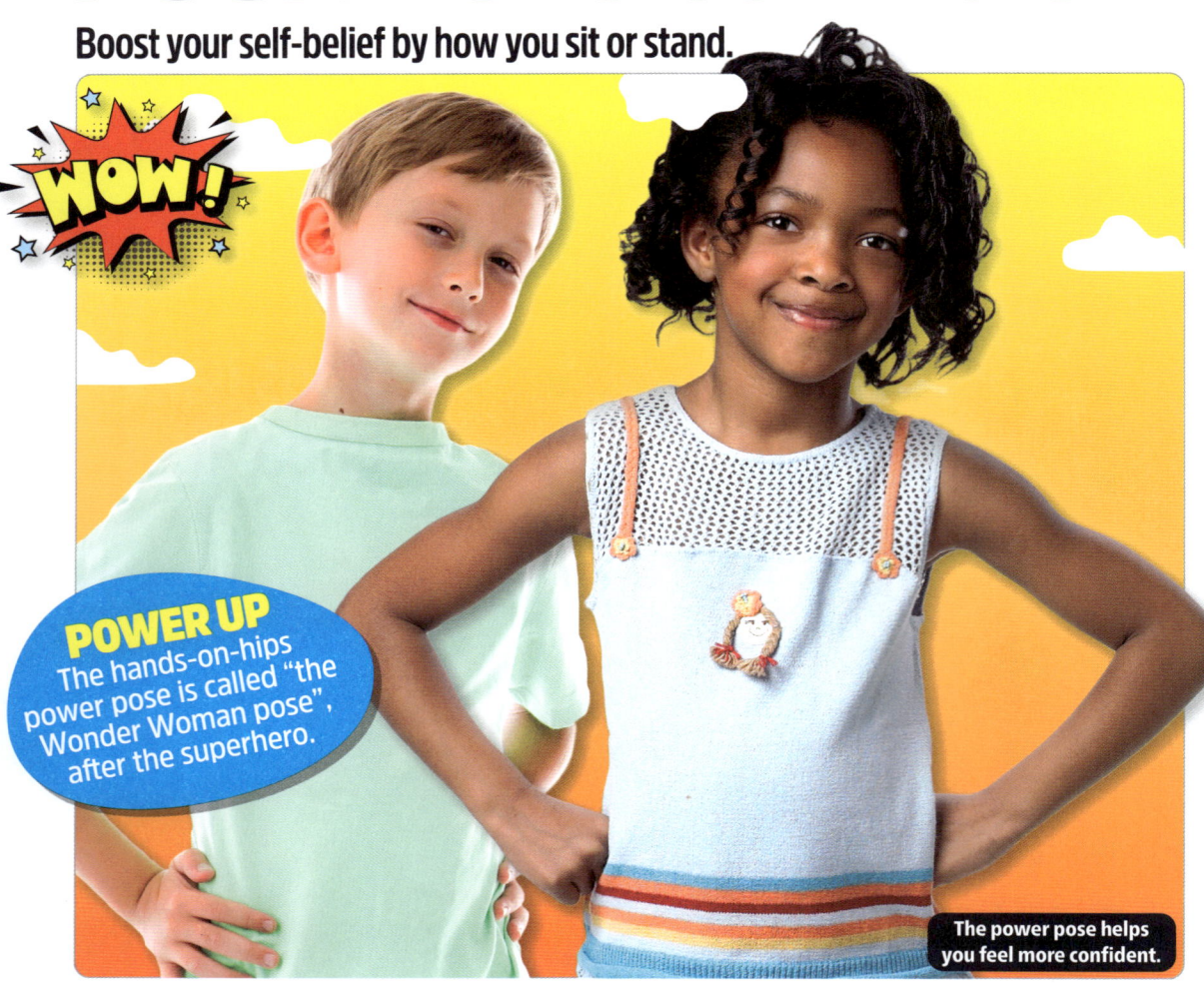

Mental wellbeing

Feel more confident

Boost your self-belief by how you sit or stand.

POWER UP
The hands-on-hips power pose is called "the Wonder Woman pose", after the superhero.

The power pose helps you feel more confident.

Being confident isn't just about what you know or think; confidence comes from how you feel in your body too.

How you hold yourself matters
How you sit or stand – your posture – influences how you feel. If your shoulders are hunched, your head's down and you're slouching, you feel differently to the way you feel when you're sitting or standing straight with your head up and your shoulders back. Try it for yourself – sit or stand slumped forward and notice how you feel. Then move your body to being more upright with your arms by your side and looking forwards. How do you feel now?

Your body talks to your brain
Research has found that when you're hunched with your arms and legs crossed, and looking down, your body releases chemicals that can make you feel more stressed or worried.

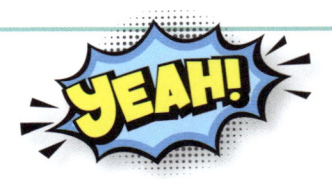

Sitting straight helps you feel strong.

Young people's coach Maria Evans says your body and brain are connected. "When you stand with your back tall, legs apart, hands on hips and chin up, your body sends the message to your mind that you feel confident and strong."

Your body language doesn't just affect how you feel, it tells other people how nervous or brave you feel too. Think about someone you see as confident: how do they carry themselves? Bring to mind a movie or TV character you admire for being brave or strong and picture how they sit, stand or walk. See if you can do the same.

Take a power pose
If you're feeling nervous, that makes you nervous, try to keep your shoulders down and your head up to help you keep the confident feeling. Evans suggests doing a power pose for a few minutes before school. "Notice how it makes you feel and how your mood has changed and become more positive."

Focus your mind

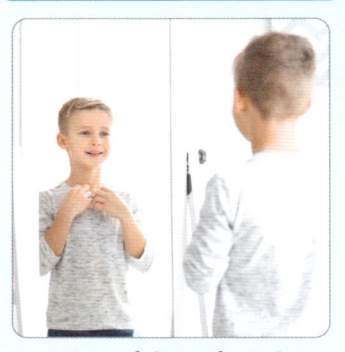

Young people's coach Maria Evans says that when you're doing something challenging, notice the negative voices in your head. "Imagine scrunching those thoughts up like paper and putting them in the bin. Are you left with supportive thoughts? If not, think of some thoughts that cheer you on. Using a mantra (a repeated phrase that helps concentration) like 'I believe in myself', in your head or out loud, can change the way you think about what you can do."

"I squeeze my hands"

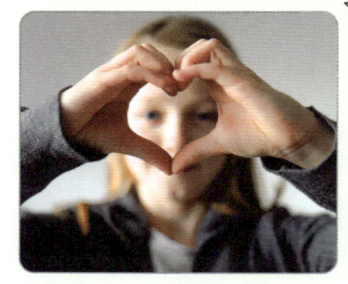

"When I feel nervous I think about all the people I have around me supporting me. I also take a deep breath and remind myself that it doesn't really matter if I say or do something wrong, as long as I do my best. I sometimes squeeze my hands together and imagine it's one of my friends, or Mummy or Daddy squeezing it and saying, 'You're doing great,' and that really helps too."
Carys, aged nine

Feel more confident

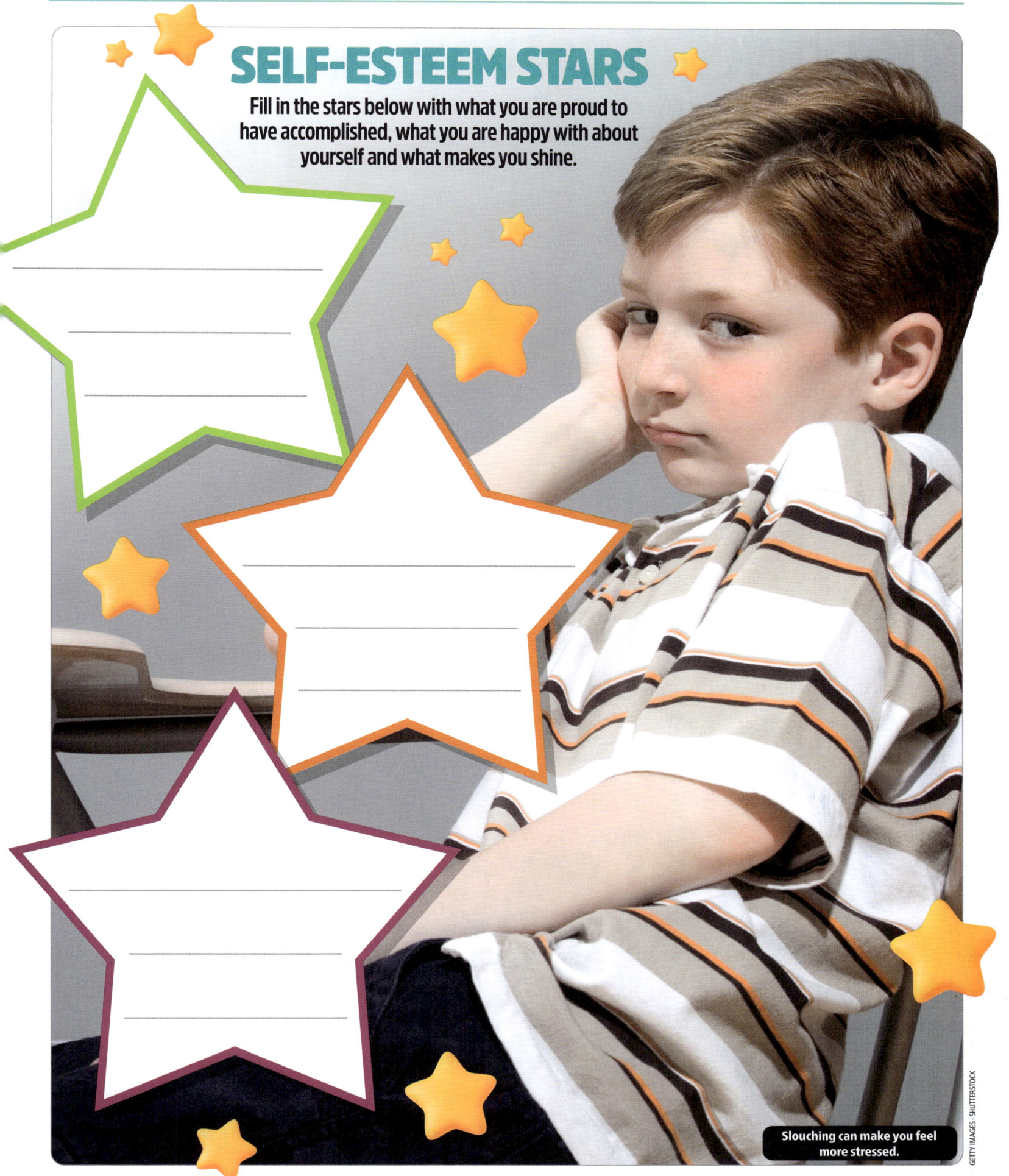

SELF-ESTEEM STARS

Fill in the stars below with what you are proud to have accomplished, what you are happy with about yourself and what makes you shine.

Slouching can make you feel more stressed.

Mental wellbeing

The power of positive thinking

Being optimistic can boost your health and pave the way for success.

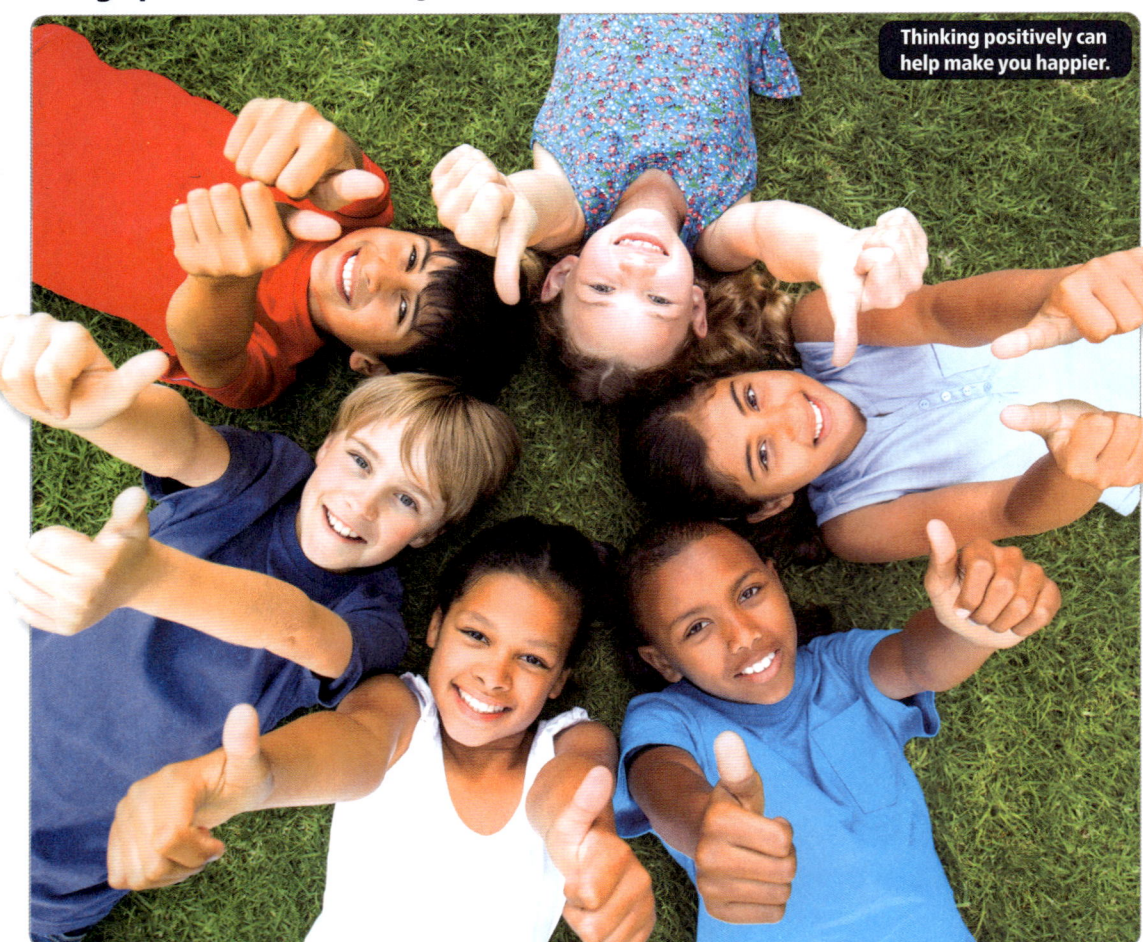

Thinking positively can help make you happier.

Is your glass of milk half-full or half-empty? This saying is often used to test people's outlook in a situation; do they focus on the positives (a half-full glass) or the negatives (a half-empty one)? Thinking positively, with a belief that most things will turn out well, is called optimism – and it's known to boost your wellbeing. The good news is that everybody can learn to think more positively.

Why is thinking positively good for you?

Research shows that people who are optimistic and think positively tend to experience less stress and cope well when faced with life's challenges. People who are more pessimistic (expect that the worst will happen) may find it hard to believe that these challenges will pass. Scientists have even found that thinking positively can make you live longer. According to Professor Tali Sharot, being optimistic about the future can make you happier and more successful. This is because you believe your goals are achievable and within reach, which encourages you to work towards them.

Try to imagine positive outcomes.

Worrying is like a fire alarm

Everybody can worry from time to time. Worrying can help to keep you safe – if you were never worried and were overly positive about how things would turn out, you wouldn't recognise risks. "Worrying is our brain warning us that there might be something threatening. It's like a fire alarm," says child psychotherapist Rachel Melville-Thomas. "The trouble is that sometimes it goes off when there isn't a huge danger to face." When this happens, you can feel anxious and hopeless about what lies ahead.

Learn to think positively

Optimism is shaped by your genes, which carry characteristics inherited from your parents, and by what happens to you. However, no matter your starting point, everyone can learn to become more optimistic. Research has shown that it can help to draw or write an outcome that's positive – for example, an image of you playing guitar, having passed your next grade. Imagining this can motivate you to work to achieve it, such as practising every day after school.

Being hopeful

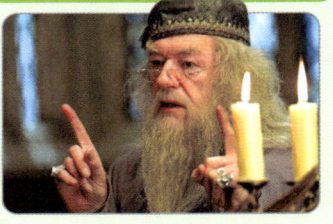

These inspirational quotes are taken from which children's books? (You'll find answers on the side of the page.)

1. "Well, maybe it started that way. As a dream, but doesn't everything?"

2. "Happiness can be found even in the darkest times, if one only remembers to turn on the light."

3. "I am not afraid of storms, for I am learning how to sail my ship."

How do I turn the "fire alarm" down?

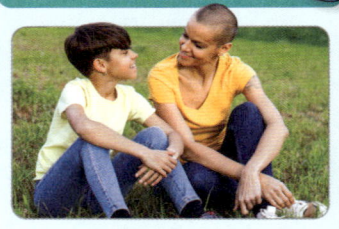

Child psychotherapist Rachel Melville-Thomas has these tips:

- Stop and see what that fire alarm is doing. Go somewhere quiet and have a think. Take five deep breaths and think of your favourite person or animal. What would they say?

- Sometimes the alarm will stop if you sing to yourself, listen to music, cuddle the cat, have a bath or have something to eat or drink. Be kind to yourself.

- Talk to a friend or trusted adult about your worries and try to understand where they are coming from.

Answers: 1. *James and the Giant Peach*, Roald Dahl. 2. *Harry Potter and the Prisoner of Azkaban*, J.K. Rowling. 3. *Little Women*, Louisa May Alcott.

The power of positive thinking

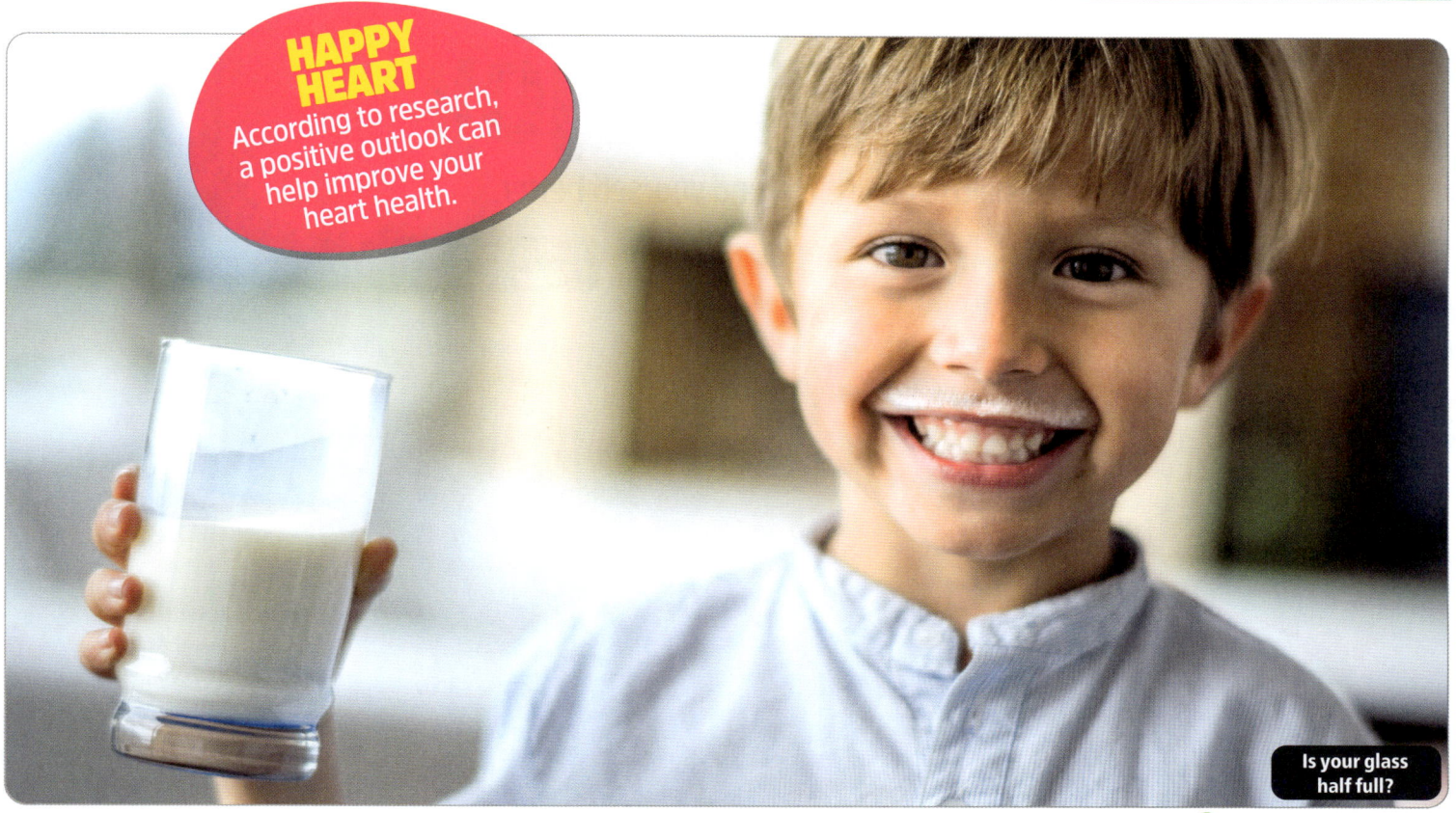

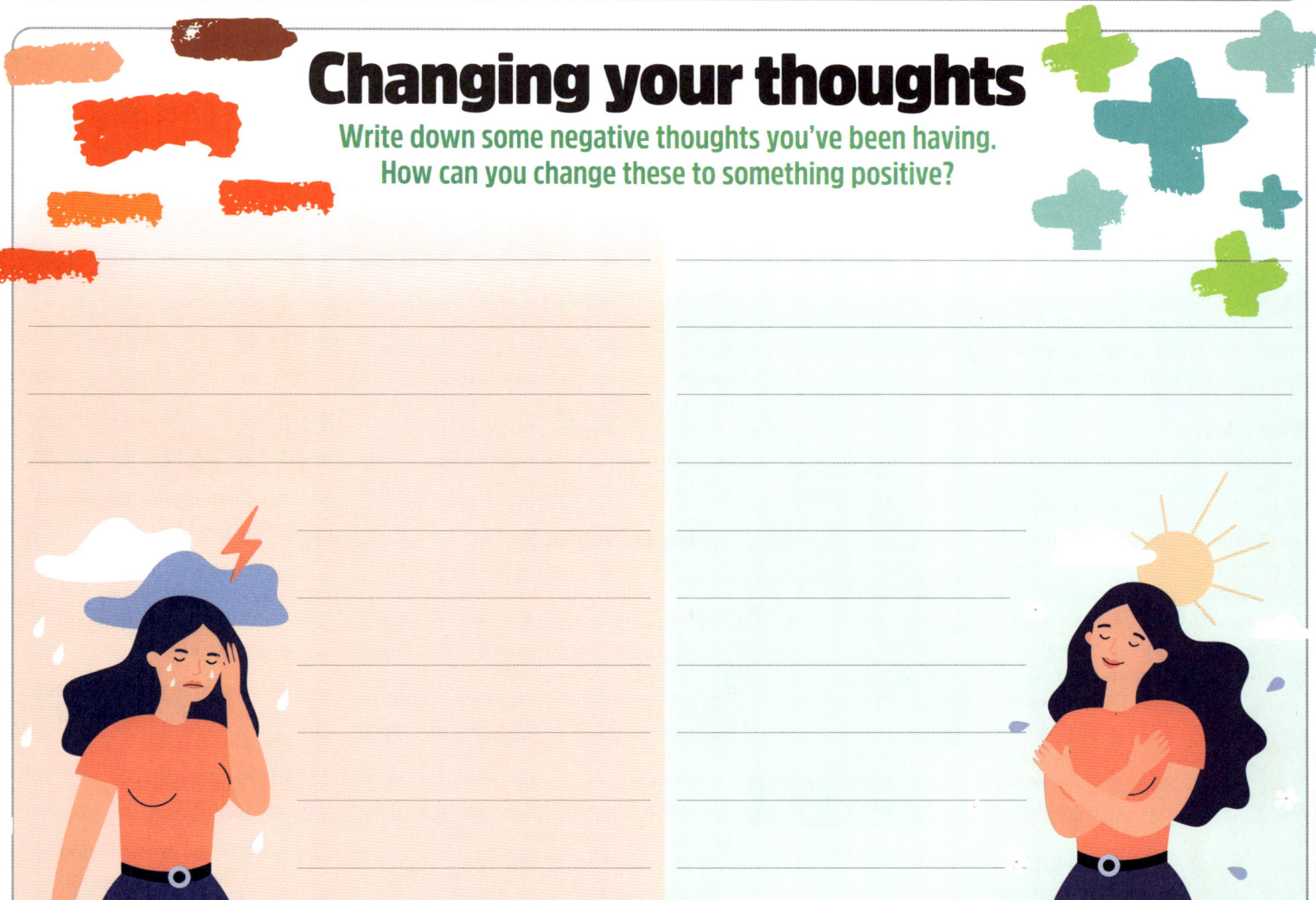

HAPPY HEART
According to research, a positive outlook can help improve your heart health.

Is your glass half full?

Changing your thoughts

Write down some negative thoughts you've been having. How can you change these to something positive?

Mental wellbeing

Fill yourself with joy

Learning how to lift your mood helps you understand yourself better.

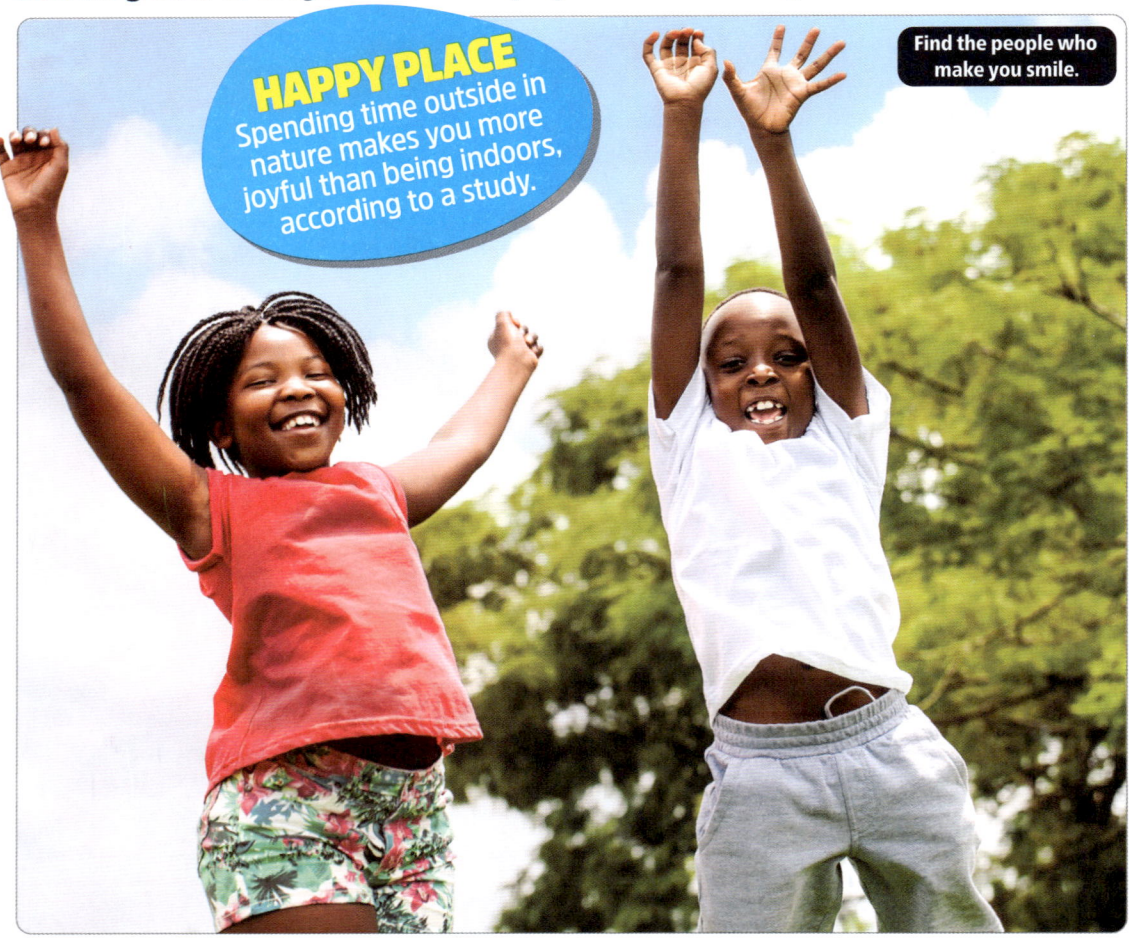

HAPPY PLACE Spending time outside in nature makes you more joyful than being indoors, according to a study.

Find the people who make you smile.

Rose says she finds joy with her cousin.

Does your heart feel lighter when you cuddle a pet or do you get a happy tingle when your favourite song is played? Joy is a feeling that comes from inside and lifts your mood – even when things aren't going your way.

What is joy?
Joy is a kind of happiness that doesn't depend on what's going on around you. It means looking forward to a picnic even though it's raining, or feeling excited about watching your favourite football team when you know they probably won't win. Joy means something different to everyone.

You could find joy by diving into a swimming pool or watching seeds grow. The Week Junior reader Rose, aged nine, says, "Joy makes me laugh and be happy, like when I'm trampolining with my cousin."

Why joy matters
Joy is like a tank of happiness you store inside yourself, ready for when you need a boost. Discovering where you find joy helps you to understand yourself better. Tal Ben-Shahar, an author and happiness expert, says this is because you face up to other feelings along the way, including anger and sadness. It means "giving yourself permission to be human," he says. When you've had a difficult day at school, you might know that curling up on the sofa to watch a film or listen to music can make you feel better.

How to find your joy
Ben-Shahar recommends keeping things simple. If you're doing 10 things at once, you won't notice which one makes you happy. "There can be too much of a good thing," he says, "and when it comes to happiness, less is often more." Focus on being positive. Studies show that paying attention to good things that happen in life rewires your brain for happiness. So Ben-Shahar suggests making gratitude a habit by writing down small things you are grateful for every day. When you know where to find joy you won't need to buy something big or go somewhere amazing to make you happy.

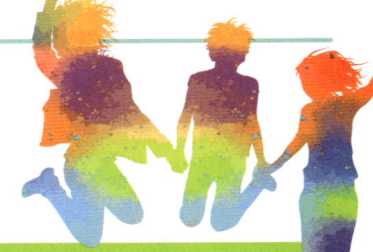

How to celebrate joy

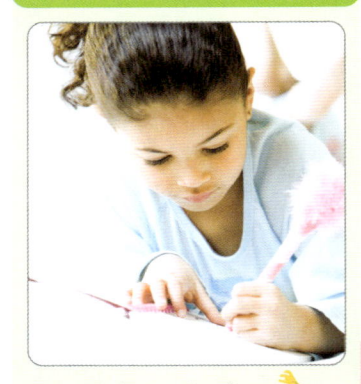

- Every day, write three good things that happened to you.
- What did people say and how did it make you feel at the time?
- Write down why you think it happened.
- Try to focus on the positive feelings it gave you.

Five tips for finding joy

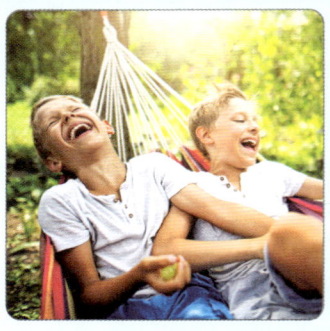

- Spend time with people who make you smile.
- Listen to your own voice; you don't have to like exactly the same things as everyone else.
- Stick to what you believe is important and fair, even if people disagree.
- Don't be afraid to try something new.
- Look for joy in small things, like silly jokes or singing funny songs.

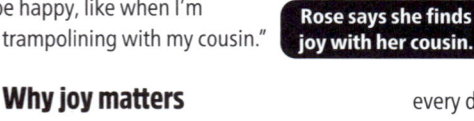

Fill yourself with joy

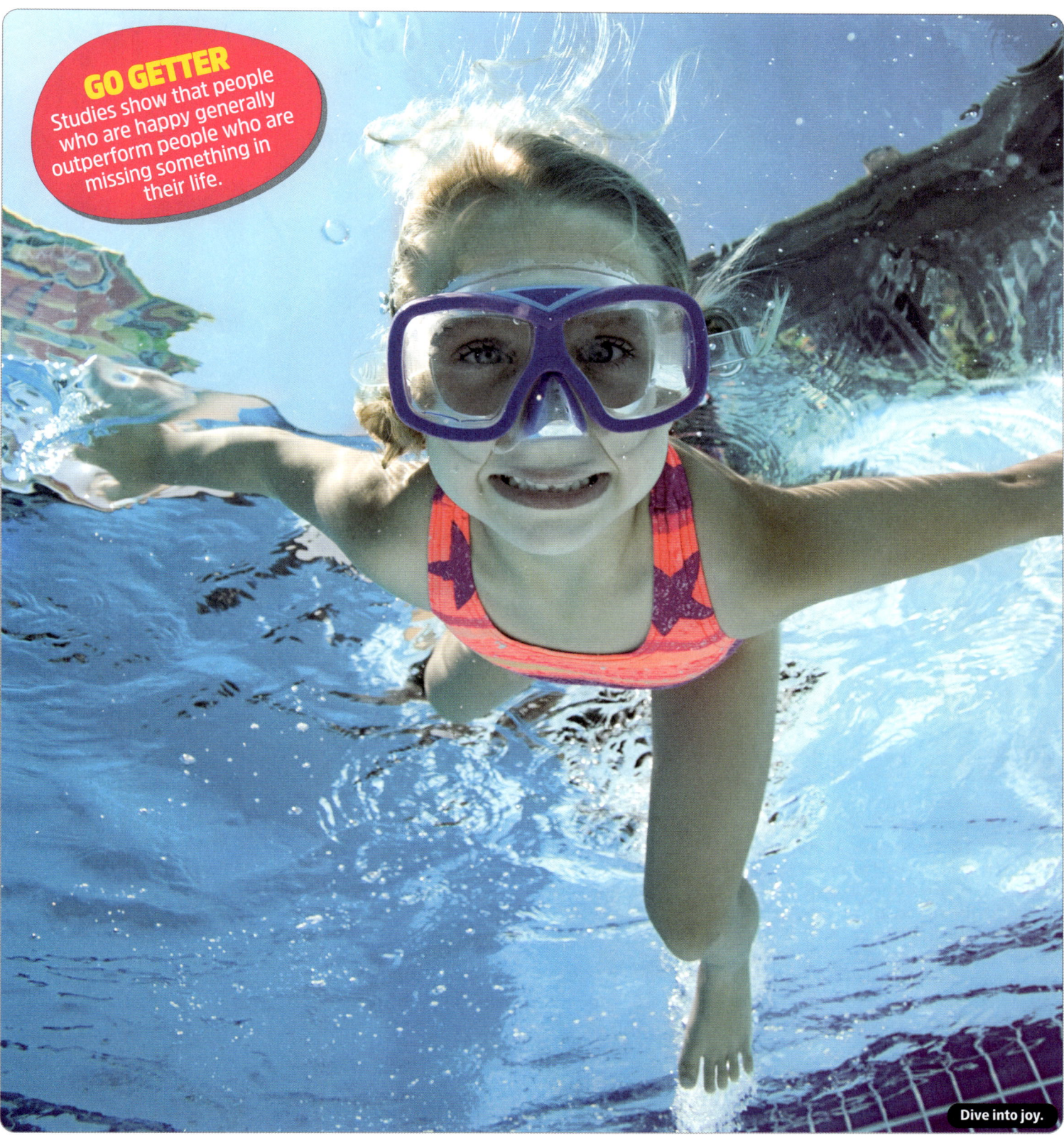

GO GETTER
Studies show that people who are happy generally outperform people who are missing something in their life.

Dive into joy.

Write down three moments of joy from your day:

_____

_____

_____

Mental wellbeing

The joy of colour

Surrounding yourself with your favourite colours can boost your wellbeing.

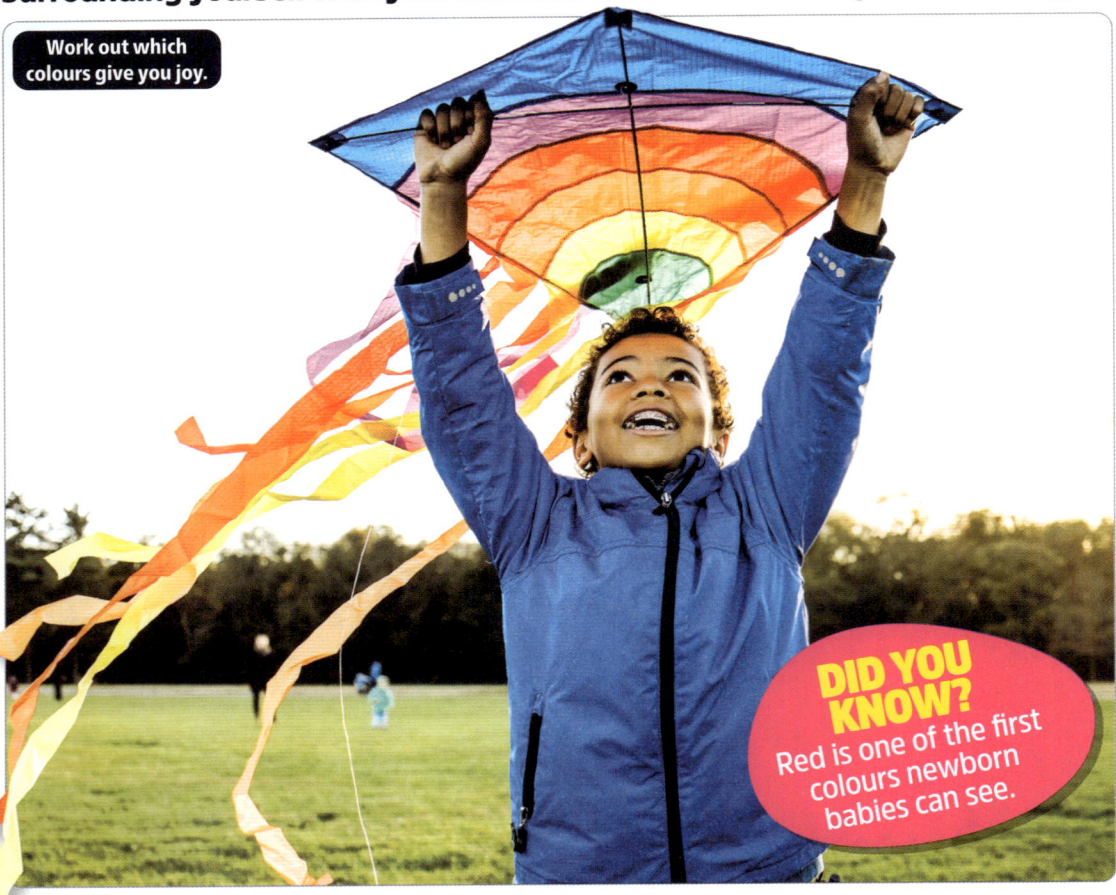

Work out which colours give you joy.

DID YOU KNOW? Red is one of the first colours newborn babies can see.

Have you ever found yourself pining for a juicy red apple? Do you feel refreshed when you walk through a green forest in spring? Or perhaps you've taken a photo of a beautiful sunset while on holiday? We are surrounded by different colours and often take them for granted – but they are linked to experiences, feelings and memories. Finding the shades that make you happy and bringing these into your life can boost your wellbeing, especially during the dark winter months.

The benefits of colour

"Colour is a way to express yourself," says colour expert Karen Haller. Whether it's your clothes, hair, nails, toys or wallpaper, colour is a tool to show your personality. "We all have colours that make us feel happy," explains Haller, who believes you should surround yourself with these colours to boost your wellbeing. There are other benefits too – colours can excite or soothe people. The use of bright colours, instead of black and white, can even help you to concentrate and to remember information more easily.

Which colour pencils do you prefer?

What colours can help to improve my mood?

Your colour likes and dislikes are personal and there's no right or wrong answer when it comes to choosing your favourite colours, says Haller. Research has shown that your attitude to colour is linked to your emotions and experiences – for example, many people love the colour blue because it reminds them of the sea. To work out which colours spark joy in you, Haller recommends pulling out all your colouring pencils and seeing which ones you like best – or think which colours you use the most.

How colour helps wellbeing

Once you've worked out the colours you find uplifting, choose how you'd like to add these into your life. Perhaps it's in your artwork or your choice of clothes or the colour of your bedroom. You could pay more attention to these positive colours when you're out and about, or create a colourful mood board to look at if you're not feeling your best. Haller suggests choosing a special object made up of your favourite colours, so you can look at it whenever your mood is a bit low.

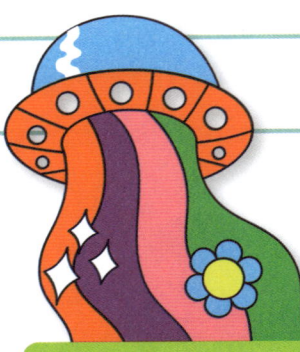

What is colour?

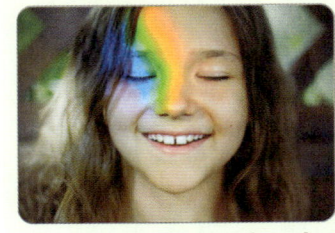

Each colour has a wavelength. The colour red has the longest wavelength and violet has the shortest. When light hits an object, the colour we see is the wavelength it reflects. So a lemon reflects yellow light, but absorbs the other colours of the rainbow. If all the colours are absorbed, that's when we see black.

Mood and colour

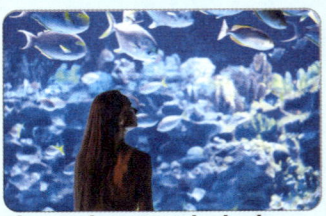

The Week Junior asked colour expert Karen Haller to describe the feel-good qualities of different colours.

- **Red**
  Energy. Helps to excite and motivate you.

- **Orange**
  Playfulness. Represents fun.

- **Yellow**
  Hope. Welcoming and warm – like sunshine. It helps you to think positively.

- **Green**
  Safety. Linked to nature, can help you feel safe.

- **Light blue**
  Calm. Helps calm your mind.

- **Dark blue**
  Focus. Can help you to concentrate.

The joy of colour

Mood board

Fill in your colour mood board by writing in or sticking in ideas for decorating your room to tell your parents.

Colours that would make me happy in my room:

What theme would I like? (Planets, animals, sport)

Ideas for my bed, walls, game storage:

Mental wellbeing

Make a colourful wind spinner

These wind spinners are beautiful moving shapes that will twirl around in the breeze. All you need to do is cut out a series of simple card strips and string them together, creating a curve or spiral.

Wind spinners make pretty and mesmerising decorations for the garden – they can even help scare the birds off a vegetable patch. You can hang one indoors, too; just put it near a window so it can turn in the breeze.

You can make different shapes.

CRAZY NAME
Another name for a wind spinner is a whirligig.

WARNING! Take care when using a needle.

What you need
- Corrugated card from a box
- A ruler
- A pencil
- Scissors
- Paints
- A thick needle
- String or wool
- Glue

TOP TIPS
Thread beads at the top or bottom as an extra decoration.

It's easier to twist and stick the strips into a curved shape with the wind spinner hanging up.

The wind spinner shape can be adapted with strips in different sizes, all the same size, or with the edges trimmed diagonally.

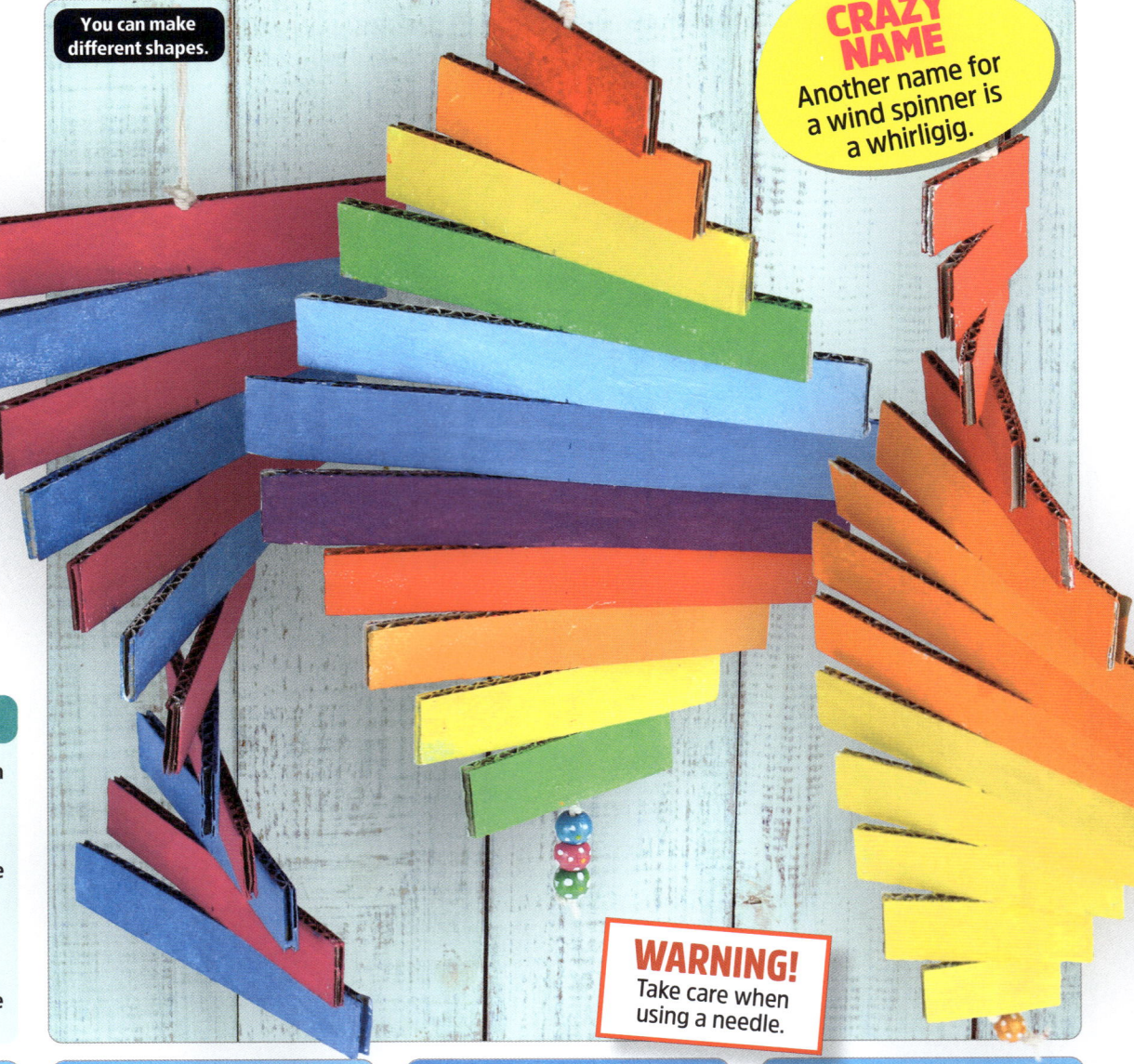

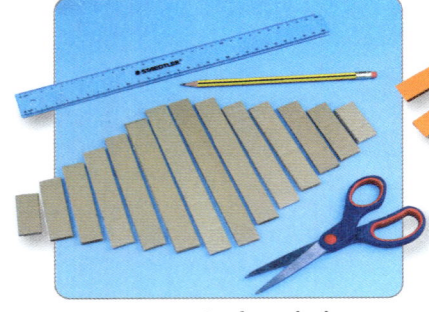

1 Cut some strips from the box card. They need to be 2cm (0.8in) wide and different lengths. You will need to cut two strips for each of these lengths. Cut it so that the corrugated holes are visible along the long edges – you'll need them there in step 3.

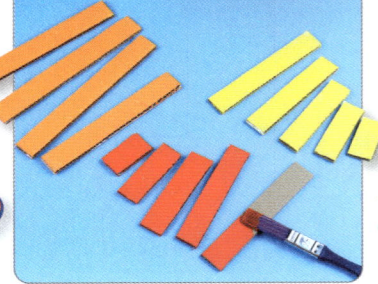

2 Paint all the strips on one side, leave to dry, then paint the other side. Leave the strips to fully dry before the next stage, too. The colours will look brighter if you have a layer of white paint underneath. When the white is dry, brush or sponge the colours over the top.

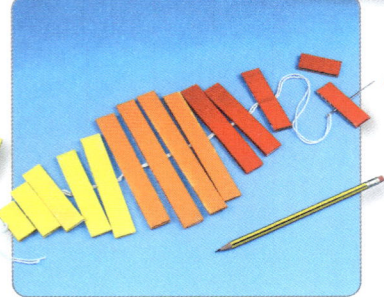

3 Mark the middle of each length of card in pencil. Thread a thick needle with a piece of string or wool 80–100cm (31-39in) long. Make a knot at the end. Thread the string through the middle corrugated hole in each cardboard strip. Leave the strips slightly spaced apart.

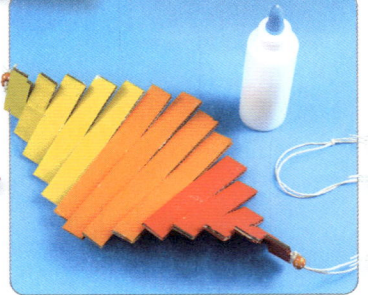

4 Dab a blob of glue in the holes around the thread. Push the strips together to make it stick in place. Make a knot at the top to fix it in place. Before the glue totally dries, turn each strip at an angle to make a twisty or curvy shape. Hang it in the wind when the glue is dry.

Head to theweekjunior.co.uk/activityhub for more crafts and recipes.

Make a colourful wind spinner

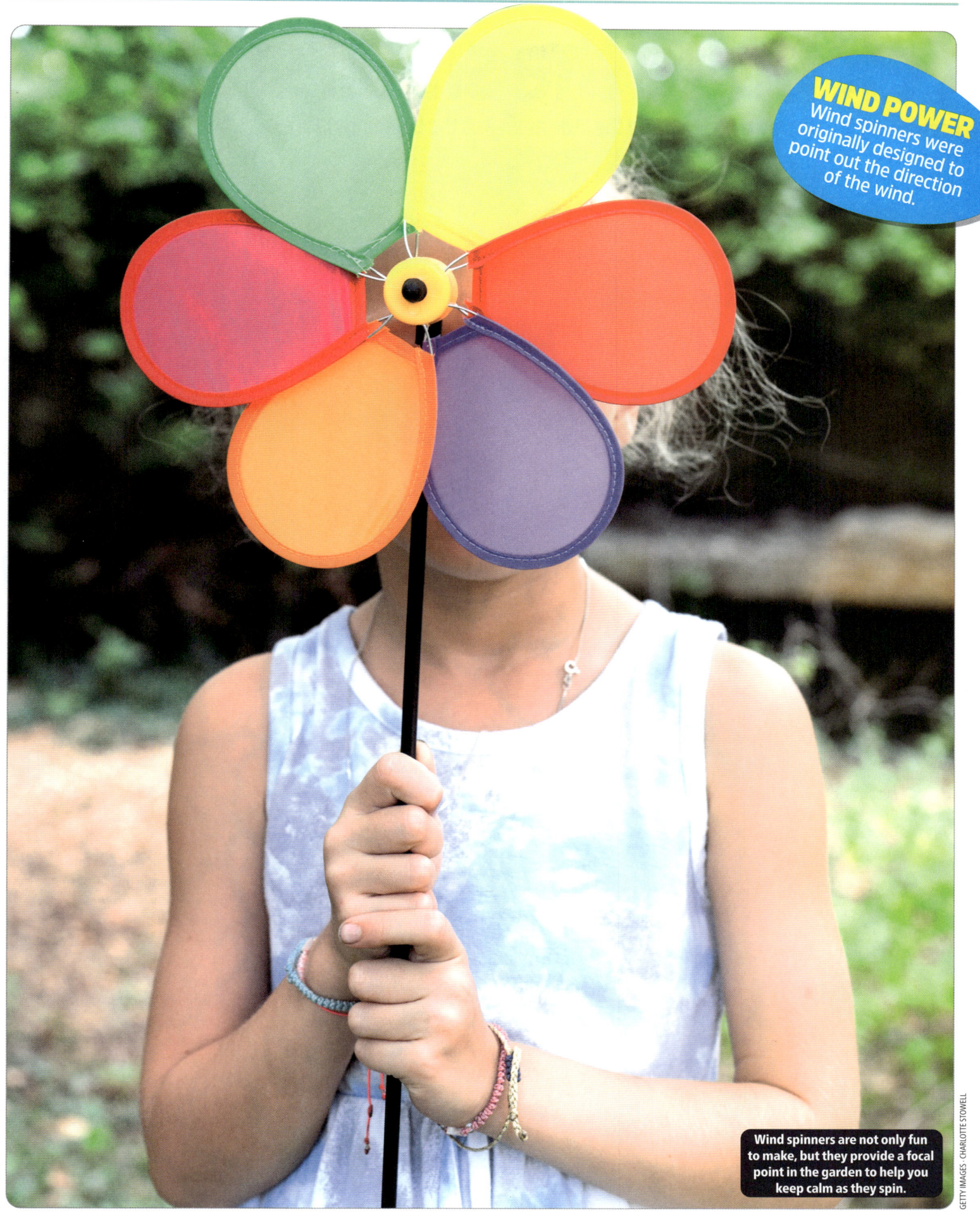

WIND POWER
Wind spinners were originally designed to point out the direction of the wind.

Wind spinners are not only fun to make, but they provide a focal point in the garden to help you keep calm as they spin.

51

Mental wellbeing

Celebrate the small stuff

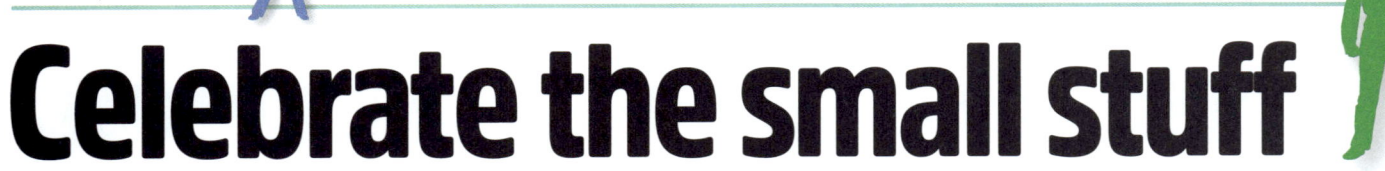

Feel more joy each day by celebrating the little as well as the big things in life.

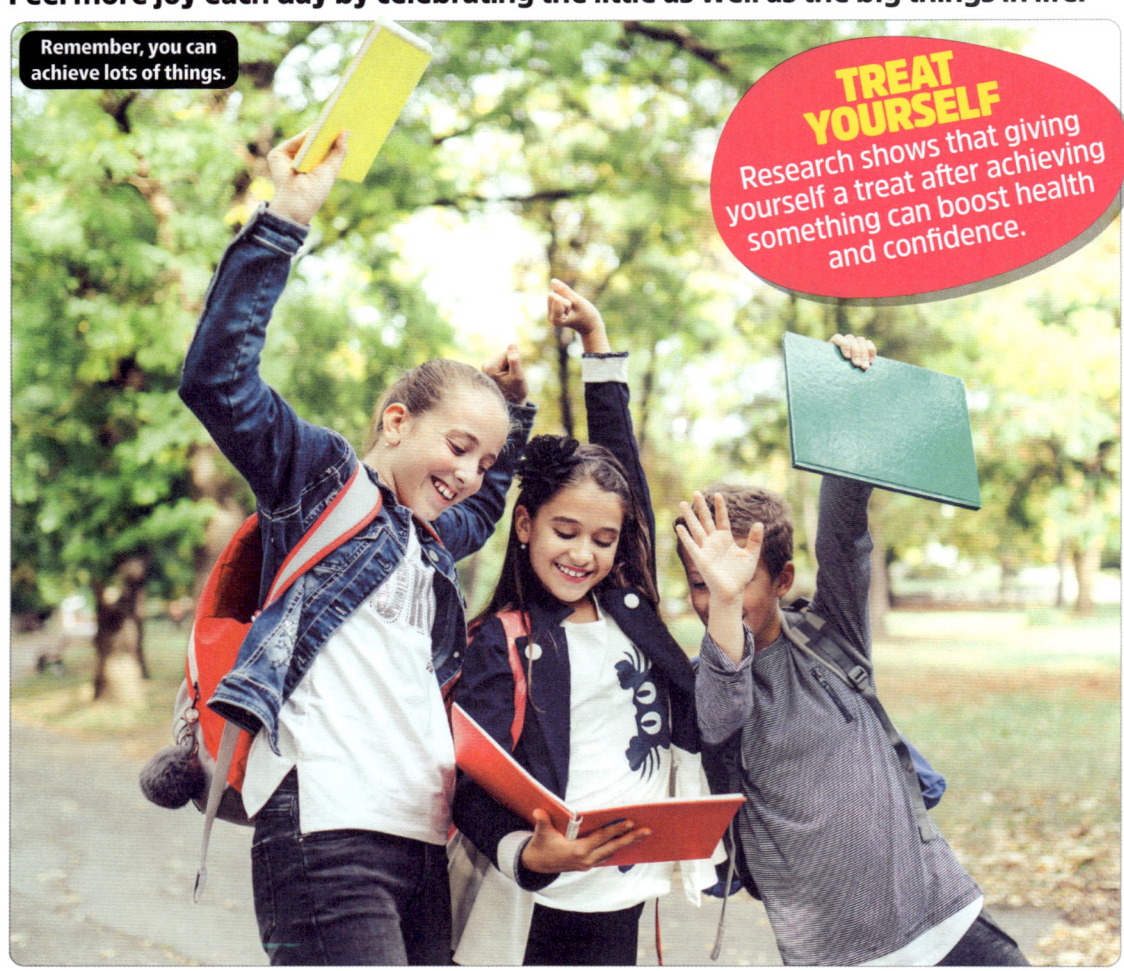

Remember, you can achieve lots of things.

TREAT YOURSELF
Research shows that giving yourself a treat after achieving something can boost health and confidence.

Big occasions and achievements are marked with fuss and fanfare but smaller moments are worth celebrating too.

Why it's good to mark moments
There are occasions that everyone celebrates, like birthdays and exam results, so it makes sense that you want to celebrate an achievement or milestone, particularly if you worked hard to get there. Celebrating is an acknowledgement of a moment that feels good, that you're proud of, or where you overcame a challenge. By celebrating you make it more memorable. This gives you happy memories to look back on and remind you of how capable you are. Francesca Geens, creator of *The HappySelf Journal*, believes it's important to mark moments. "Celebrating helps your brain release chemicals like dopamine so you learn that it feels good to put in the effort in the first place. This boosts your confidence in your abilities to do difficult thingsor take on challenges, and it builds your resilience."

Celebrate by doing something fun.

Noticing the little wins in life
Humans naturally focus on and remember the negatives rather than the positives. This is why you remember when you get something wrong more than when you do something right. It means you need to make extra effort to notice when things – even small things – go well.

Celebrate the small stuff
Think about how pleased you feel when you've tidied your messy bedroom, finished a puzzling piece of homework or kept your cool when something annoyed you. You feel a sense of accomplishment. By taking a moment to celebrate, you acknowledge your achievement and capabilities. You'll feel good and remember it the next time you're faced with a messy bedroom, difficult school work or a tricky situation. Celebrating doesn't need to be a big deal. It can be telling someone else about it, doing something fun like dancing around your room, or saying out loud to yourself, "That was not easy, but I did it!".

Look for the positives

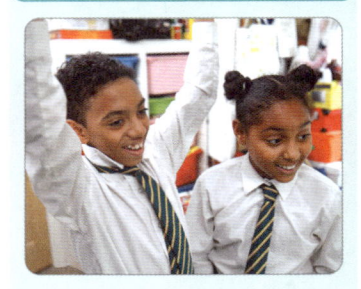

Francesca Geens, creator of *The HappySelf Journal*, says when you practise noticing good things in your day, or take time to celebrate your wins, it helps your brain to look for the positives. "The more you do this, the more your brain gets better at seeing good things around you, the more feel-good chemicals get released and the more resilient you become. This helps when you face stressful situations."

"Rewarding myself helps to motivate me"

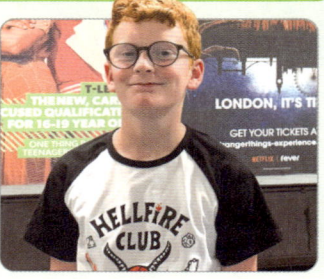

"I hate homework so much that it can ruin my day, but if I get a really difficult piece of homework done, sometimes I celebrate, as it's an achievement. Making a plan about how I'm going to reward myself for finishing it helps to motivate me, like something nice to eat or chilling out and watching TV. My parents celebrate my big achievements, like passing exams, but they can forget about the smaller things. It would be good if adults encouraged more acknowledgement of the smaller, everyday wins."
Sonny, aged 12

52

Celebrate the small stuff

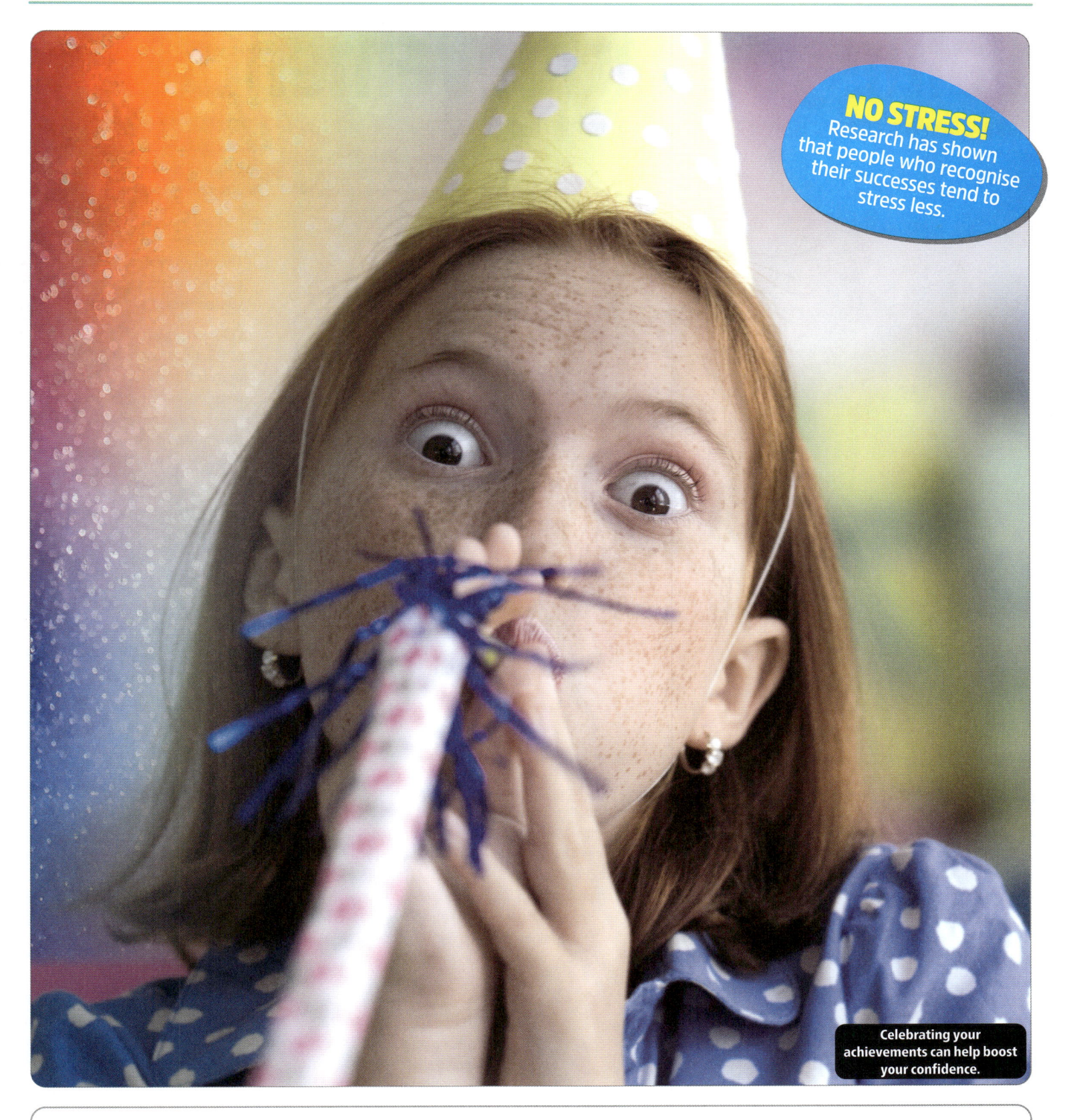

NO STRESS! Research has shown that people who recognise their successes tend to stress less.

Celebrating your achievements can help boost your confidence.

List three little things you could celebrate this week:

Mental wellbeing

Value your achievements

Making healthy comparisons can inspire you to aim high.

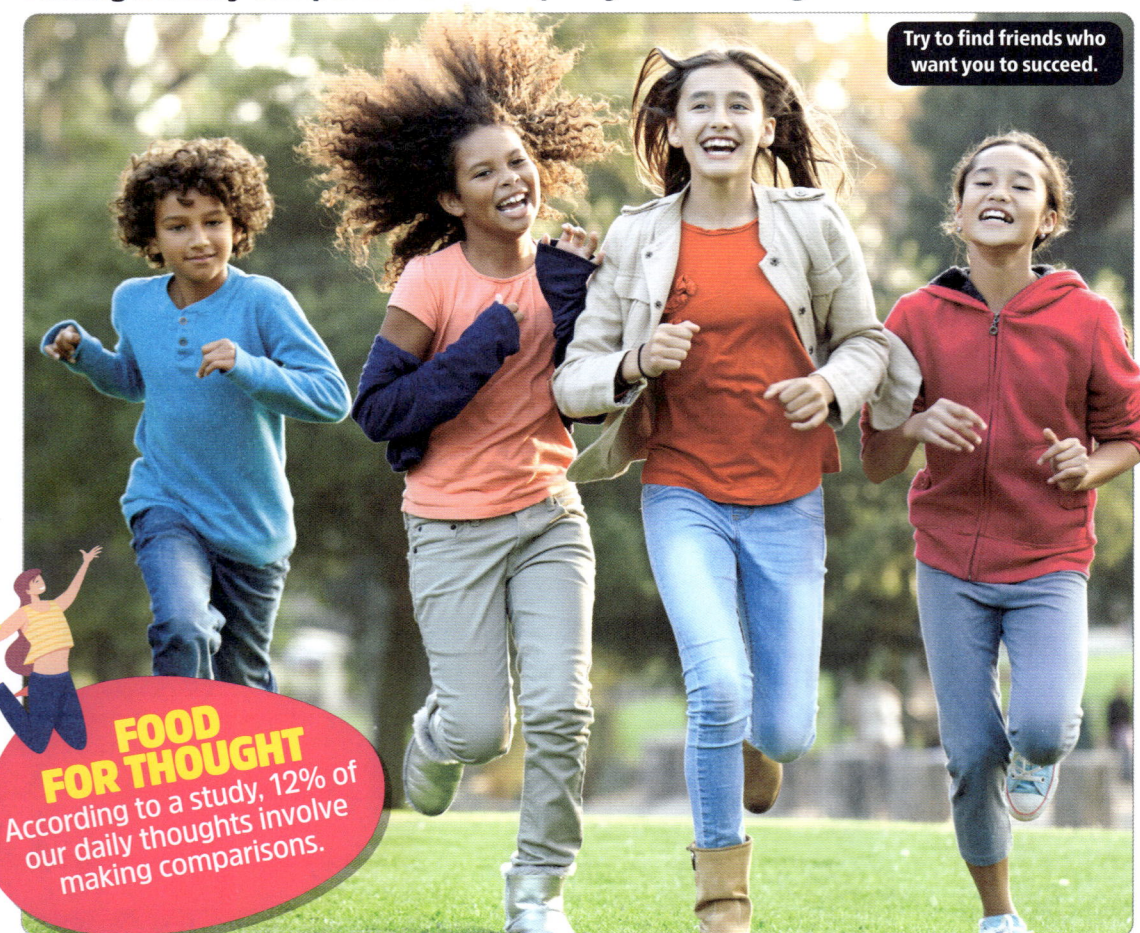

Try to find friends who want you to succeed.

FOOD FOR THOUGHT
According to a study, 12% of our daily thoughts involve making comparisons.

Do you often compare yourself to other people? Comparisons can help to make decisions and motivate you but they can also pull you into a comparison trap.

Why is it so easy to compare yourself to others?
Whether it's the number of goals you've scored at football or how many books you've read, it's easy to compare yourself to someone else. Scientists say it's a natural behaviour that helps humans learn from each other, live happily together and achieve more. Although comparing can be good for you, it's not always helpful and you can find yourself stuck in a comparison trap. This is when you always measure yourself against others and base your feelings on how well they seem to be doing.

Can comparisons be good for you?
Becky Goddard-Hill is a child therapist (someone who helps children understand their feelings) and author of Create Your Own Confidence. She tells The Week Junior that comparisons can make us feel good and bad about ourselves. "Comparing up" means seeing someone doing better than you and using that to inspire yourself to aim higher and try harder. However, Goddard-Hill says, "Sometimes it can make you feel rubbish about yourself and knock your confidence."

"Comparing down" is when you see someone who seems like they're not doing as well as you. This might make you feel you're doing well, says Goddard-Hill but it can also stop you wanting to improve.

Follow accounts that make you laugh.

Escape the comparison trap
If your feelings depend on what other people are doing, "Surround yourself with cheerleaders," suggests Goddard-Hill. Notice how people make you feel and spend time with friends who celebrate your strengths. If you follow social media accounts that make you feel you are failing in any way, unfollow them. "Find ones that make you laugh or show you lovely places instead," she says. Finally, focus on your own achievements and how you can improve. "The best person you can compete with is yourself," says Goddard-Hill.

Positive comparisons
Top tips for making positive, healthy comparisons.

- Instead of trying to be the best, aim to be your best. This means you value your own achievements and not someone else's.
- Celebrate progress instead of the final result. It doesn't matter if someone is better or faster than you, it's how hard you try that's important.
- Set some goals and track your progress. Instead of saying "I can't do it", say "I can't do it yet".

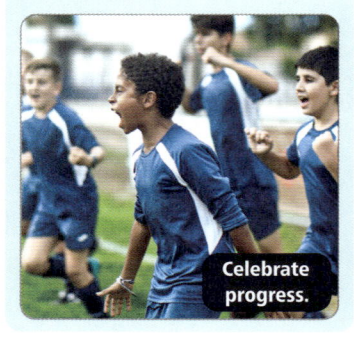

Celebrate progress.

"I could play like that one day too"

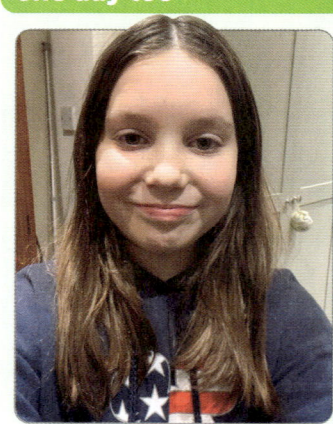

"Watching the Lionesses win the Euros last summer showed me how well girls can play football. It made me think I could play like that one day too."
May, aged 11

Value your achievements

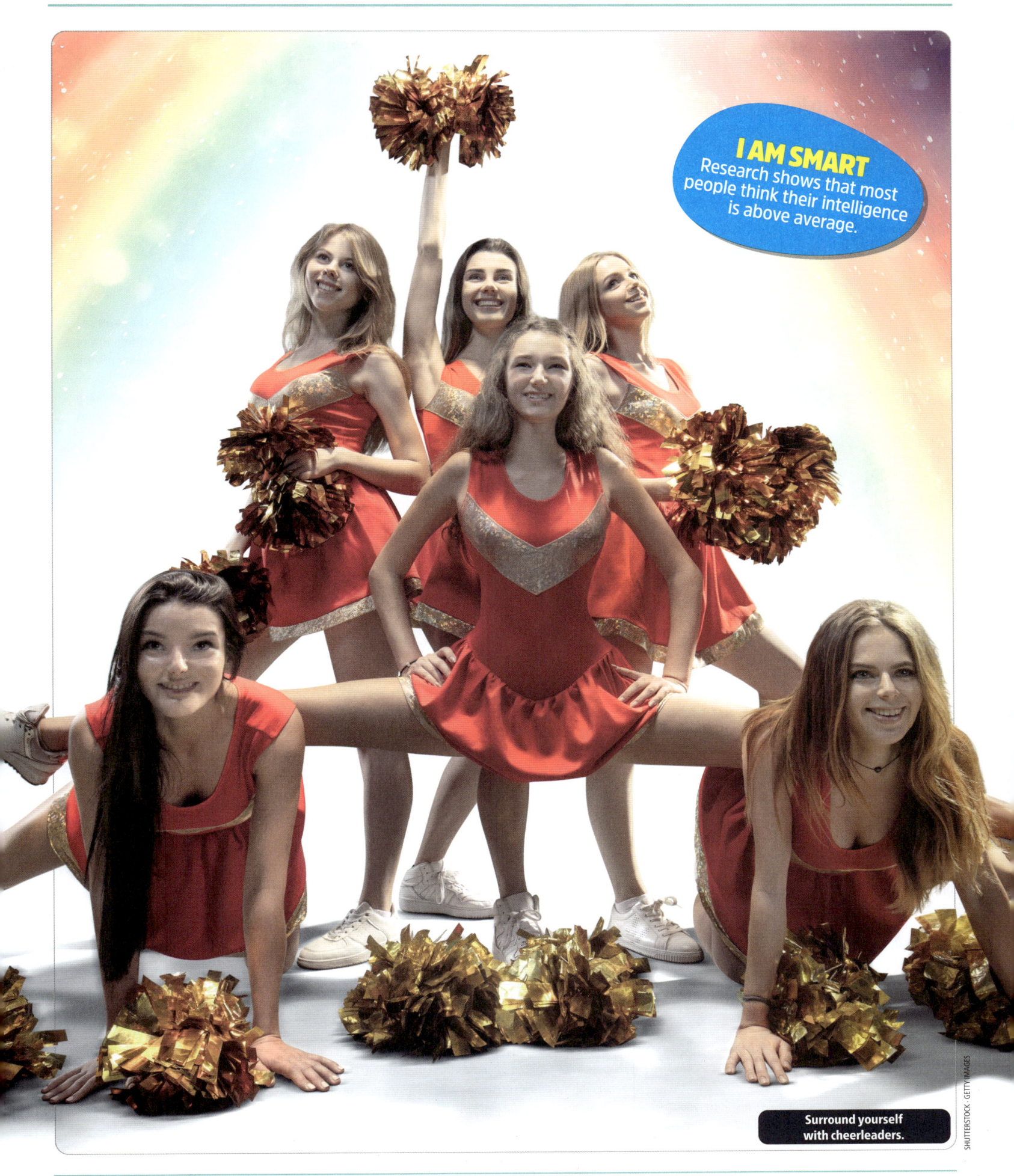

I AM SMART
Research shows that most people think their intelligence is above average.

Surround yourself with cheerleaders.

55

Mental wellbeing

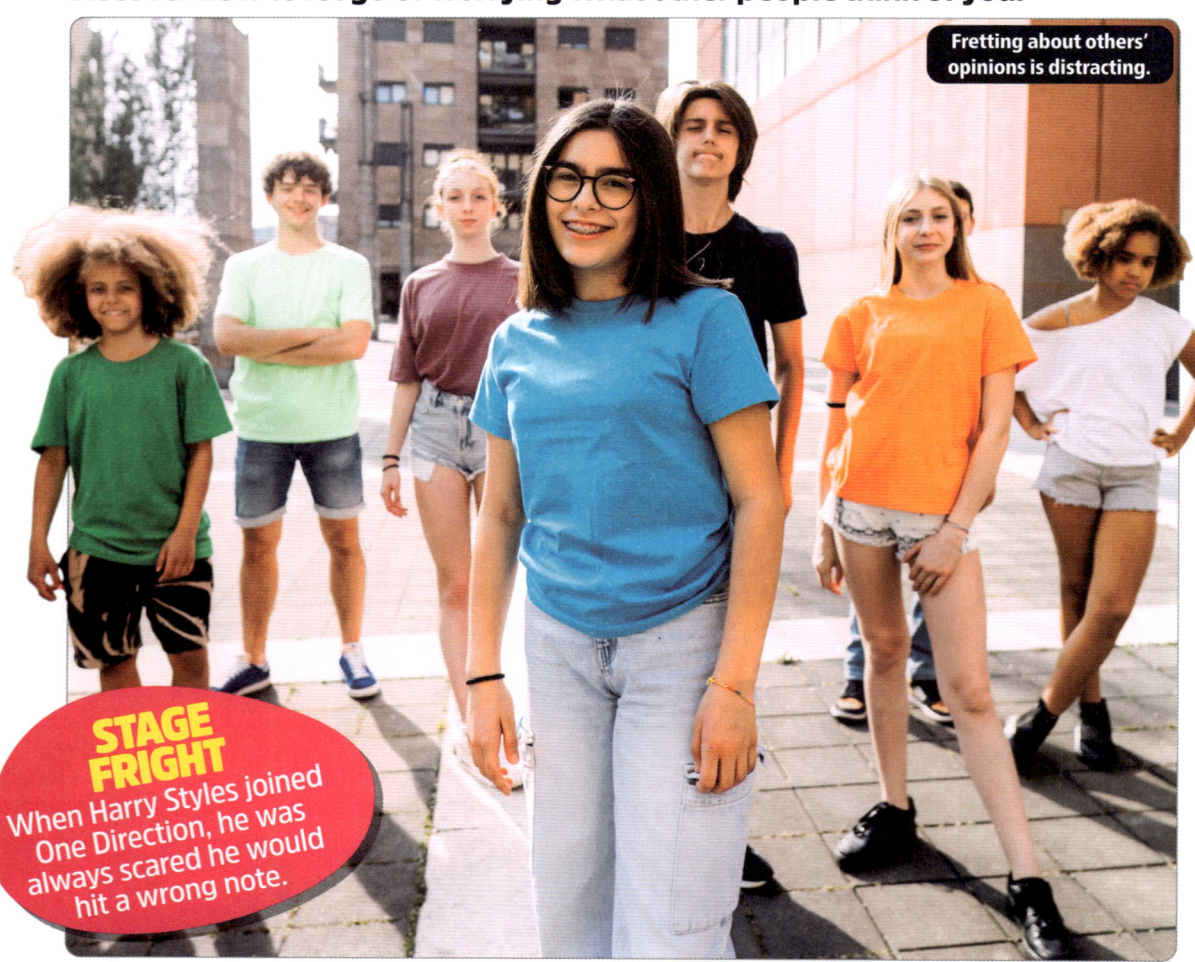

Stop caring what others think
Discover how to let go of worrying what other people think of you.

Fretting about others' opinions is distracting.

STAGE FRIGHT
When Harry Styles joined One Direction, he was always scared he would hit a wrong note.

When you're worrying what other people might be thinking of you, what you're doing or how you look, it distracts you and can stop you from being yourself.

Are people thinking about you?
There are many situations where you might imagine other people are forming an opinion of you. If you're giving a presentation in class, performing on stage or taking part in sport, it's natural that people are going to look at you. However, there may be other times when you think others are looking at you, even though you are not doing anything to draw attention – when you're walking down the street, for example, chatting to your friends or just sitting quietly reading. If you assume that others are criticising you, it can lead to worrying.

The effects of worrying
When you worry about other people's opinions, you spend a lot of time guessing what they are thinking about you. Doing this distracts you from what you're doing – like schoolwork, a conversation or a game you're playing. This can stop you from doing the things you want or need because you imagine other people might think you are doing it wrong or that you look silly. Young people's coach Maria Evans explains that worrying what other people think can mean you act in a way that isn't a true reflection of you. "Worrying about what people think can distract you and you can get caught up in impressing or pleasing other people at the expense of what feels true to you."

Spend time with friends who know you.

How to worry less
It isn't possible to know what someone is thinking about you, or even if they're thinking of you at all. Evans says you cannot control other people's thoughts, no matter how hard you try. "It can be helpful to list things you can control, and focus on those instead. Reminding yourself that you are kind, brave, thoughtful and loved will help. Make plans with people who really know you and enjoy your company. It's a great way to remind yourself that there are people you can be yourself with, and how good that feels."

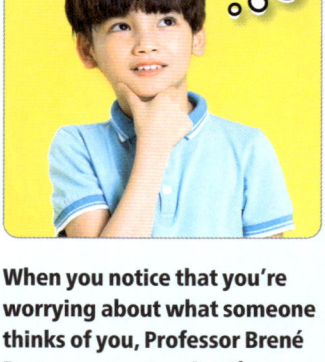

Reality check
When you notice that you're worrying about what someone thinks of you, Professor Brené Brown suggests using the words, "The story I'm making up…" before you say out loud or in your head what your worry is. For example: "The story I'm making up is they think my hair looks stupid." This should give you a reality check because it reminds you that you can only guess what someone else is thinking – you don't know for sure.

"To help me feel calm I use different techniques"

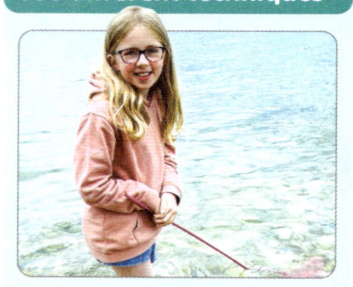

"Being the centre of attention makes me anxious. To help me feel calm, I use different techniques like my anchor – pressing my forefinger and thumb together and then thinking of something happy. Then I might give myself a hug by crossing my arms and taking a deep breath. Finally, it also helps to visualise my anxiety, give it a colour, turn it into a ball and throw it far away from me. Then I don't worry so much about what people are thinking."
Kay, aged 11

Stop caring what others think

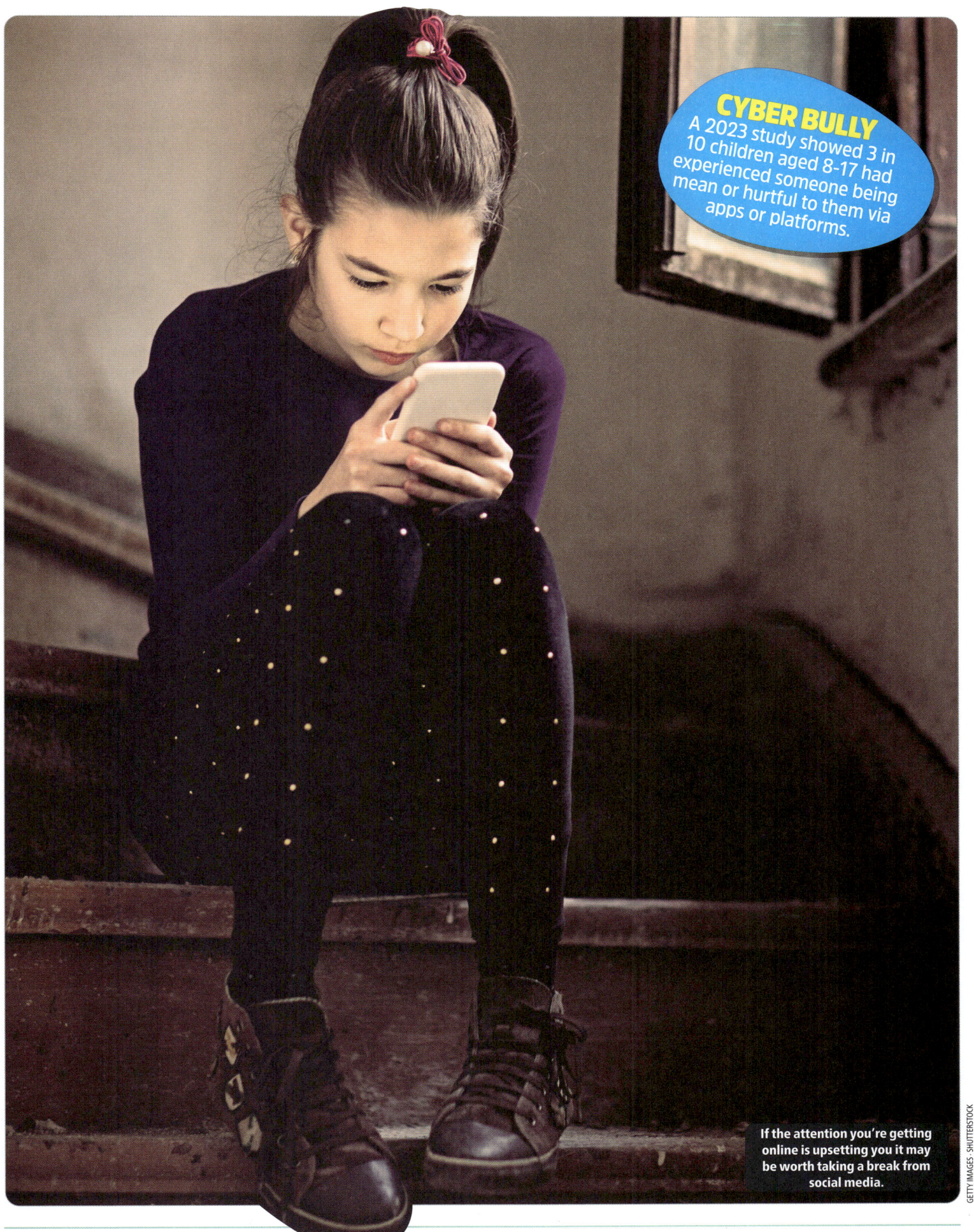

CYBER BULLY
A 2023 study showed 3 in 10 children aged 8-17 had experienced someone being mean or hurtful to them via apps or platforms.

If the attention you're getting online is upsetting you it may be worth taking a break from social media.

Mental wellbeing

The benefits of helping others

Volunteering your time and effort can boost your happiness and confidence.

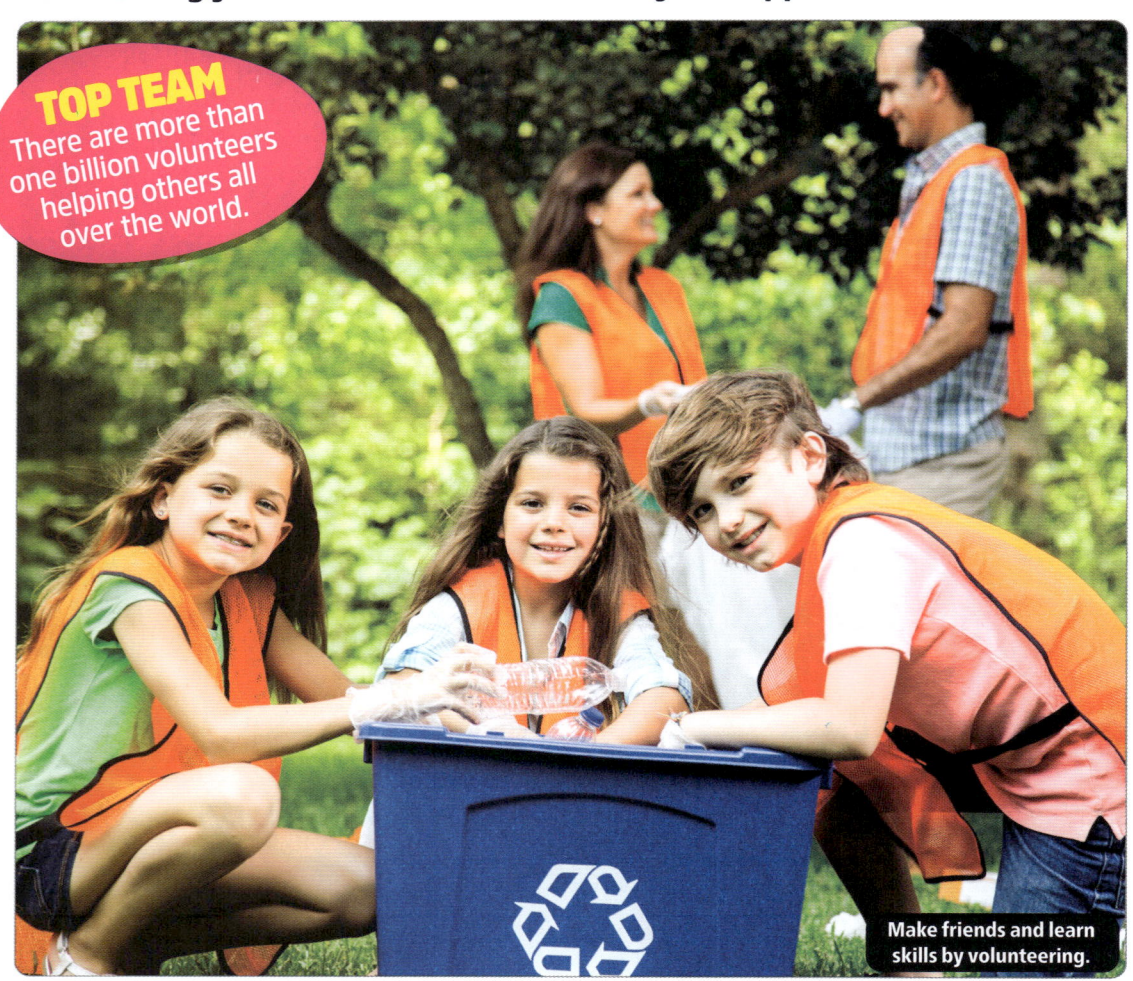

TOP TEAM
There are more than one billion volunteers helping others all over the world.

Make friends and learn skills by volunteering.

Helping others

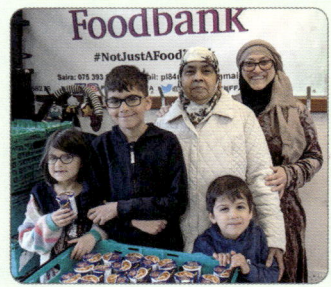

Eve, aged seven, and her brothers Kamran, 11, and Harris, four, helped out at a local food bank near their home in London. Eve said volunteering made her feel "happy to give food to people that are less fortunate than us." The experience also inspired them to raise £1,230 for the charity through a sponsored triathlon challenge.

Volunteering ideas that make a difference

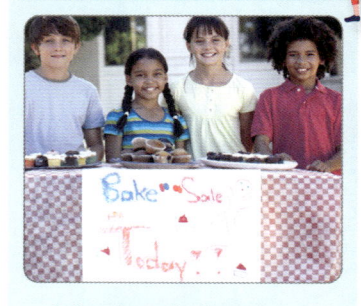

Have you ever noticed you feel good and happier after helping someone else? Volunteering isn't just great for the people or cause you support, it can boost your wellbeing too.

What is volunteering?
Volunteering means giving your time, energy or skills without expecting anything in return. Millions of people around the country volunteer every year, and there are lots of ways you can join them, including raising money for charity; helping in your local community garden or park; or even carrying a neighbour's shopping home.

How is volunteering good for me?
According to Susan Albers, a psychologist (an expert in thoughts and feelings), volunteering has been shown to reduce stress and make you feel better about your life. This is because being kind and doing things for other people activates the reward part of the brain and releases feel-good chemicals like dopamine and serotonin. Albers says that volunteering has other benefits too, such as feeling part of a community, making friends and learning skills.

Helping others feels good.

How can I become a volunteer?
There are lots of ways you can volunteer. Albers recommends finding something that is meaningful to you. If you love sport, say, then ask if your club needs help coaching younger players. If you're passionate about protecting the environment, organise a litter pick or beach clean. You could also ask at your local library, community centre or school for volunteering opportunities. Make sure you check with a parent or carer before you start, and see if friends or family want to join in. Albers says involving family or friends can be "a great way to boost your mental health. It's free. It's an activity that everyone can do. It doesn't require a lot of skill or time."

- **Join a beach clean**
  The Marine Conservation Society has a list of beach cleans around the UK on its website.

- **Write a letter**
  Exchange letters with older people in care homes who may be lonely. The National Literacy Trust's My Dear New Friend project has lots of ways to get started.

- **Raise money**
  Organise a cake or craft sale, sponsored readathon or car-washing service. Donate the money you make to your favourite charity.

The benefits of helping others

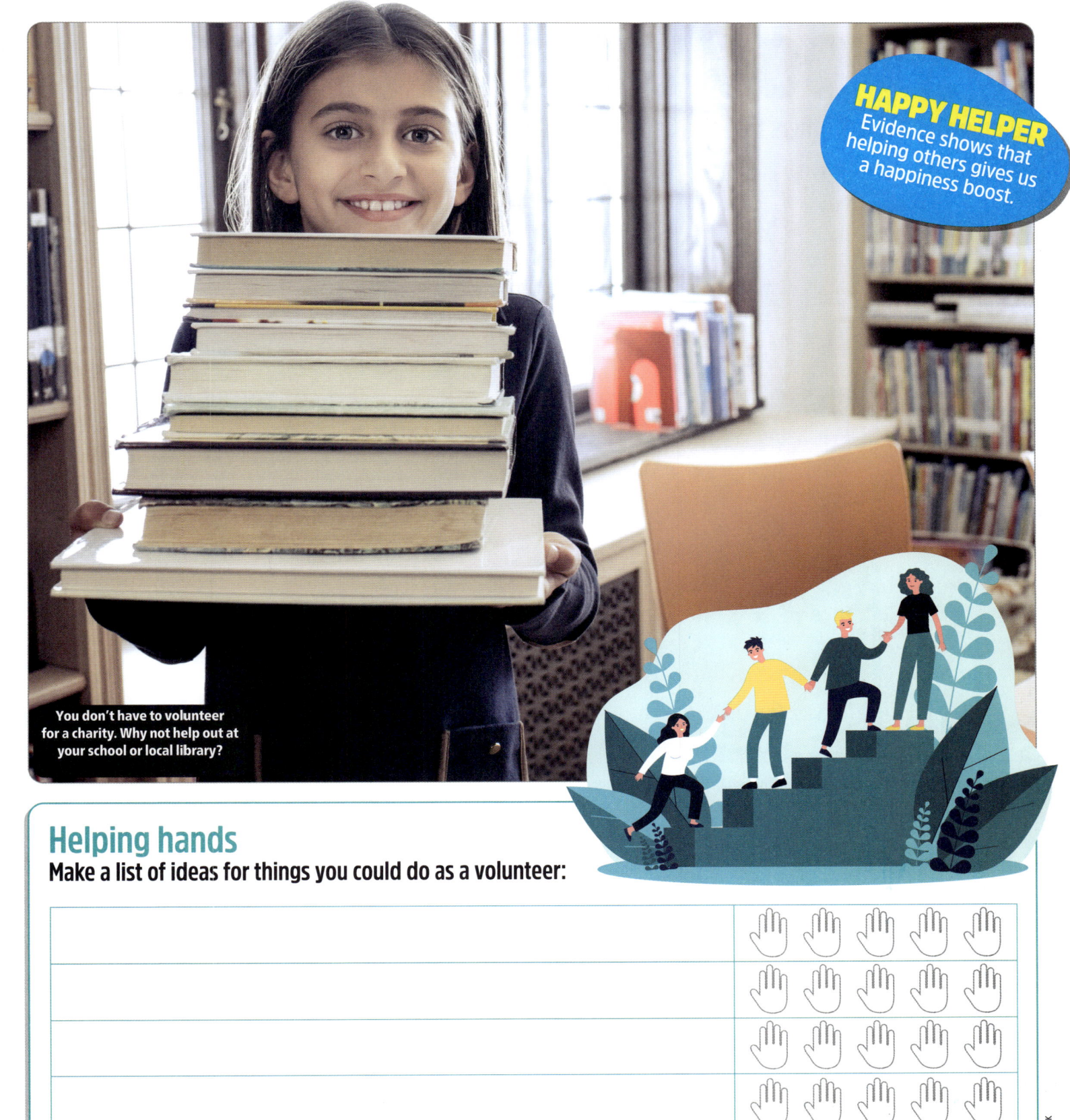

HAPPY HELPER
Evidence shows that helping others gives us a happiness boost.

You don't have to volunteer for a charity. Why not help out at your school or local library?

Helping hands
Make a list of ideas for things you could do as a volunteer:

	🖐 🖐 🖐 🖐 🖐
	🖐 🖐 🖐 🖐 🖐
	🖐 🖐 🖐 🖐 🖐
	🖐 🖐 🖐 🖐 🖐
	🖐 🖐 🖐 🖐 🖐

Once you've made a list of the different ways you could volunteer, colour in one of the hands beside the task every time you carry it out so you can see your achievement. If you need help coming up with a list, there are some ideas on the opposite page or you could visit www.royalvoluntaryservice.org.uk for more information.

59

Mental wellbeing

It's good to ask for help

Learning how to ask others to lend a hand is an important life skill.

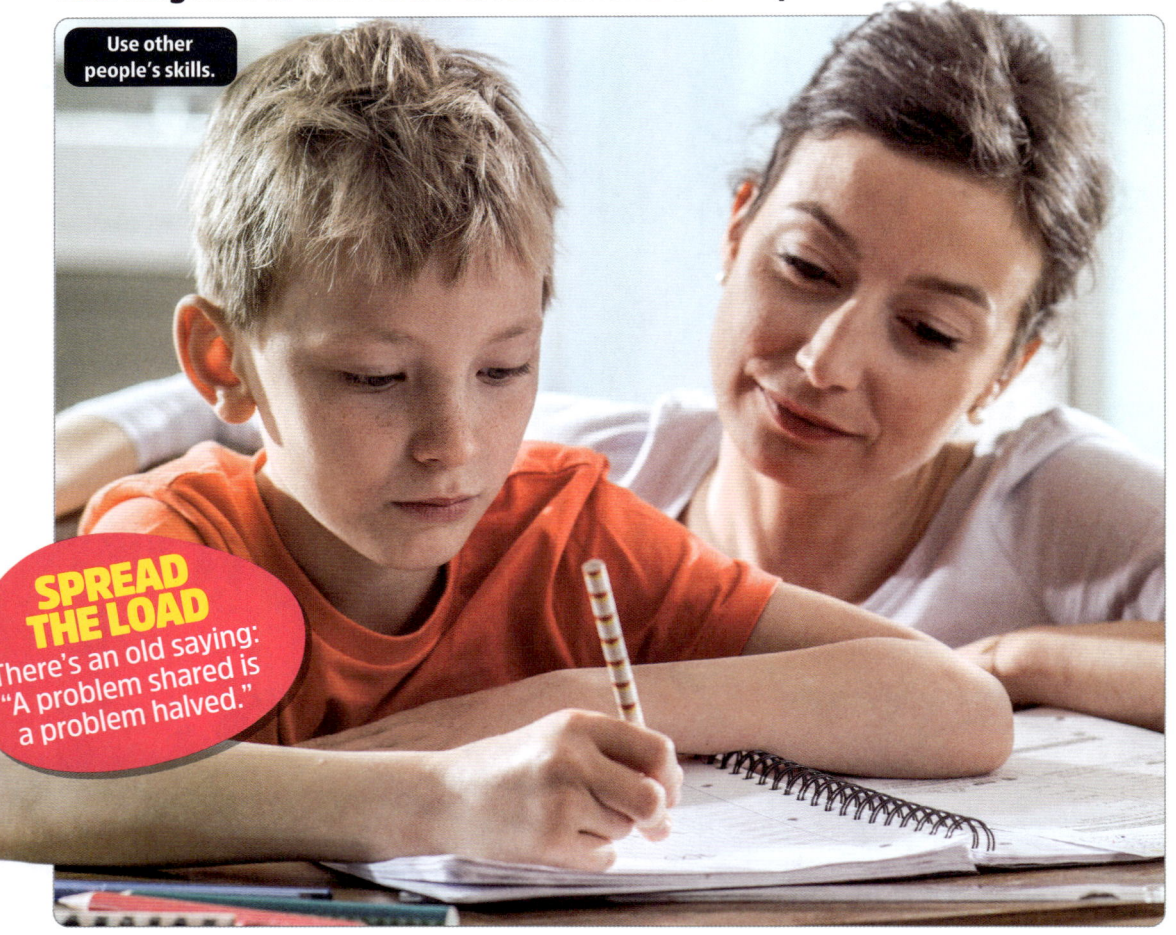

Use other people's skills.

SPREAD THE LOAD
There's an old saying: "A problem shared is a problem halved."

Ways to ask someone to give you a hand

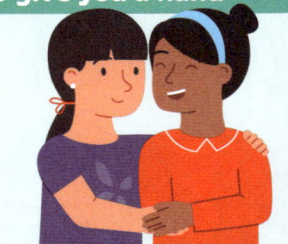

- I'm confused about this, can you explain it to me please?
- I'm finding things hard, can I talk to you about it please?
- I've tried doing it in different ways and I'm still stuck, can you help please?
- Can I take a break and then can we go through it together please?
- I want to do this myself but it might help to talk it through. Can we do that please?

"I needed help to start a piece of writing"

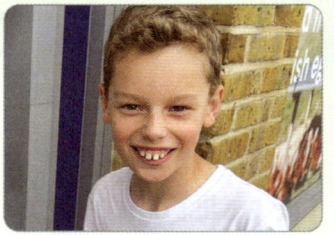

"At school I was struggling with a piece of writing in English. We were asked to write some paragraphs in the third person to describe moving to another country. I found this tricky and I thought hard about some ideas but I definitely needed help. I asked my teacher for some adjectives to get me started. At the end I thought it was one of my best pieces of work, so I was really pleased that I had asked for help!"
Noah, aged 11

Part of growing up is learning how to work things out for yourself. However, when you're feeling frustrated, confused or lost you don't have to struggle alone.

When you might need help
There are lots of reasons why you could need help, for example, with schoolwork; resolving a disagreement; learning a new skill; or when you feel sad, anxious or angry. Feeling frustrated because you're finding something difficult, or it's taking a long time to make progress, can also make you feel like you can't do it. These are all signs that you need help. When you're struggling with something but you tell yourself you should be able to do it on your own, asking for help will move you forward more quickly than trying on your own.

What stops you asking for help
Asking for help isn't always easy. It can be tricky if you're not sure who to ask. You might assume they won't want to get involved or they haven't got the time. If you're embarrassed or ashamed that you need help, or if you think asking for a helping hand is a sign of weakness, it makes it harder to turn to another person. Angela McMillan, a counsellor who advises young people, says asking for help can feel risky. "We may feel scared that it won't be taken seriously or that it isn't a big deal to the other person – or even that they won't know what to say."

Learning from others is fun.

Asking for support is brave
Everyone finds things difficult sometimes – you're not the only one. McMillan believes asking for help is an act of bravery. "Letting someone in, trusting them with your story and asking them to listen to you and help you come up with ideas of how to deal with a problem takes great courage. When you ask for help it takes the pressure off trying to figure out everything by yourself." There are other benefits too. By asking for help, you practise speaking up for yourself and saying what you need. It also shows you how someone else might feel when they're struggling, which means you could be more able to offer a helping hand when someone needs it.

It's good to ask for help

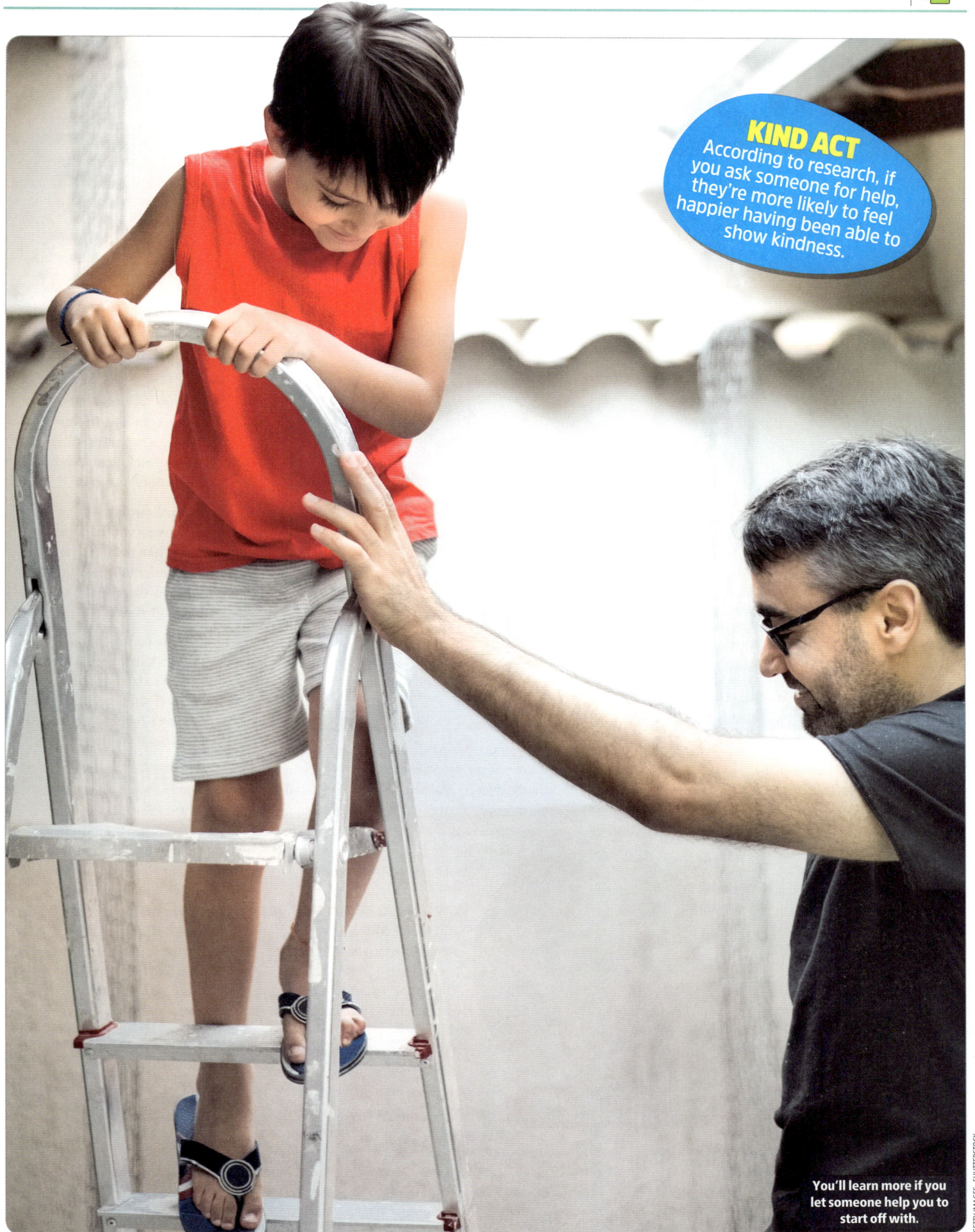

KIND ACT
According to research, if you ask someone for help, they're more likely to feel happier having been able to show kindness.

You'll learn more if you let someone help you to start off with.

Mental wellbeing

Open your mind

Being curious about the world around you can boost your confidence.

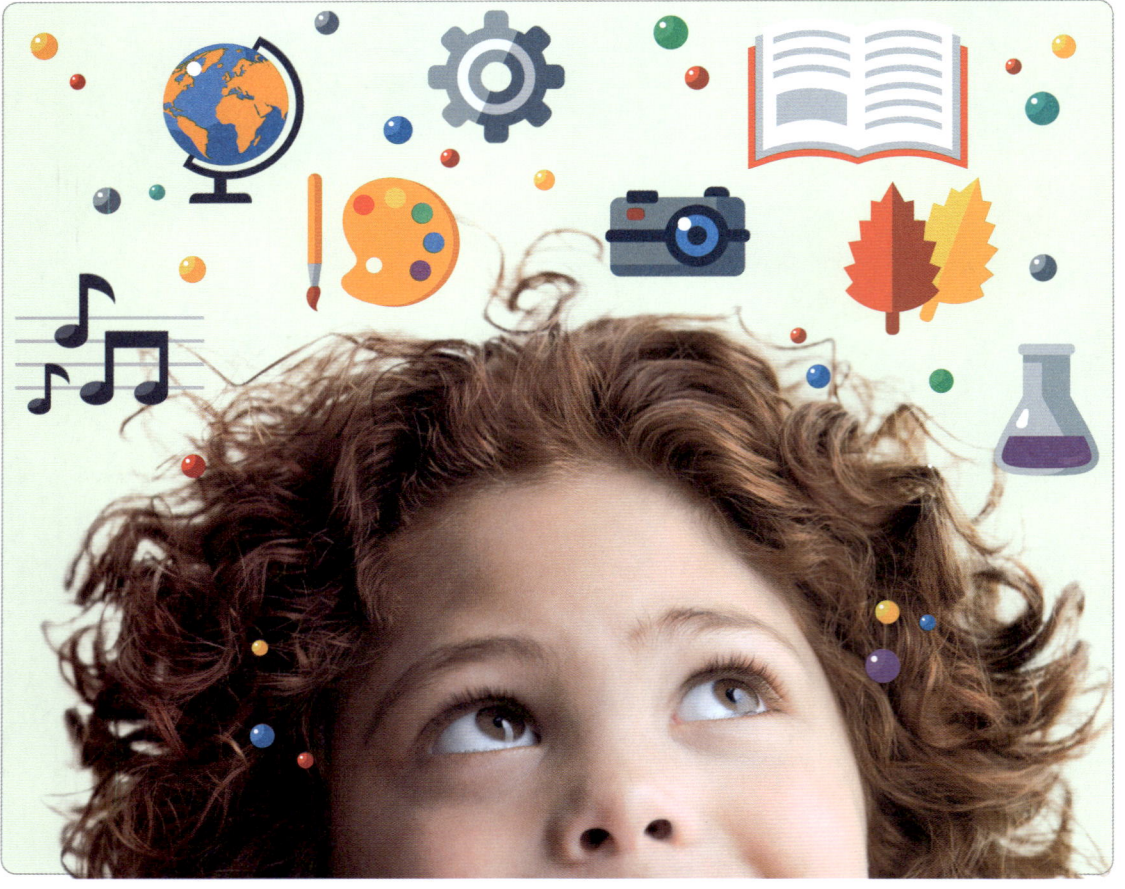

Tips for being curious and open-minded

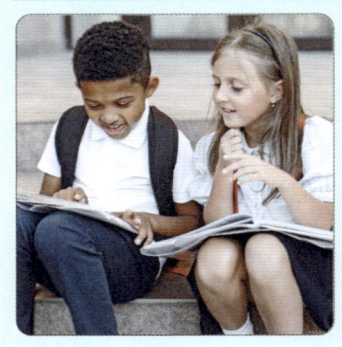

- Talk to someone in your class you haven't spoken to before and find out about their interests.
- Think about something you have a strong opinion about, like being vegetarian, and think of three reasons why someone might have a different view.
- If you're curious about a subject, learn more by talking to friends, looking in books and online. Make sure you use a reliable source; ask a teacher if you're not sure.

Opening your mind to new people and experiences will help you make friends and discover new interests. Don't worry about it – have a go!

What does having an open mind mean?
Having an open mind and being curious means trying to understand other people's thoughts and ideas, even if you don't always agree with them. It also means trying new experiences and exploring different ways of doing things. You can have an open mind about anything. A *Week Junior* reader, Elliot, who is nine, says he likes finding new ways to build LEGO. "Learning from the LEGO books inspired me to make good models by myself," he explains. The new school term means there are lots of opportunities to open your mind, find a new activity to try, make new friends and learn about yourself.

How is it good for you?
There are lots of benefits to being open-minded. Kendra Cherry is an author and expert in thoughts and feelings, and she says it helps you to learn new things about the world and the people around you. This makes you feel more confident and positive about facing challenges. Having an interest in other people gives you more empathy, which means you understand and share their feelings, says Cherry. Being open to fresh ideas can also spark exciting new ones of your own.

Elliot enjoys finding new ways to build LEGO.

How can you be more curious and open-minded?
Start by asking questions, says Cherry. So if you're unsure about joining a new club, ask yourself what's stopping you from doing it. Imagine how it feels to learn a new skill, meet new people and make new friends. Don't jump to a sudden decision but give yourself time to think about it first. If someone says something you disagree with, then instead of deciding they are wrong or arguing back, take a moment to consider why they might have that opinion. Finally, open your mind to new ideas and ways of thinking. Even if you think you are an expert on a subject there is always more you can learn, Cherry says.

Understanding bias
"Confirmation bias" is when you pay more attention to something because it agrees with your views, and ignore information that challenges them. For example, if you think cats are better than dogs, you're more likely to notice when a dog behaves badly and a cat is cute and cuddly. This can close your mind to what dogs and cats are really like.

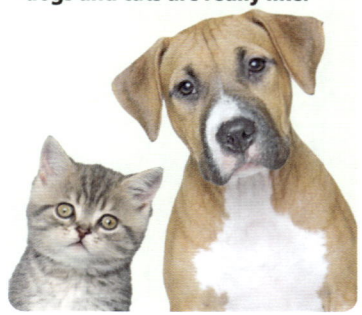

Open your mind

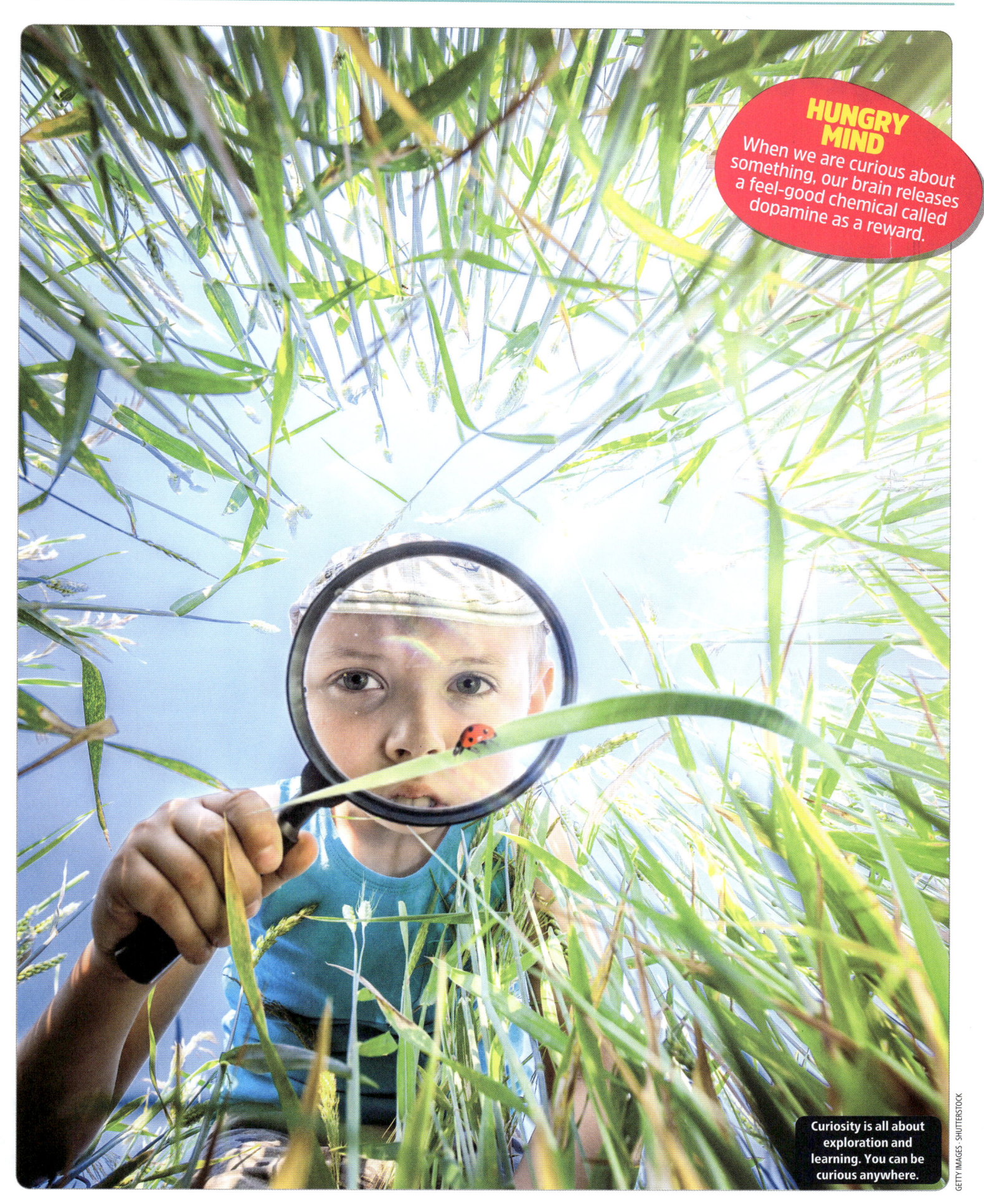

HUNGRY MIND
When we are curious about something, our brain releases a feel-good chemical called dopamine as a reward.

Curiosity is all about exploration and learning. You can be curious anywhere.

Mental wellbeing

Enjoy the great outdoors

Paying attention to the sights and sounds of nature is good for your wellbeing.

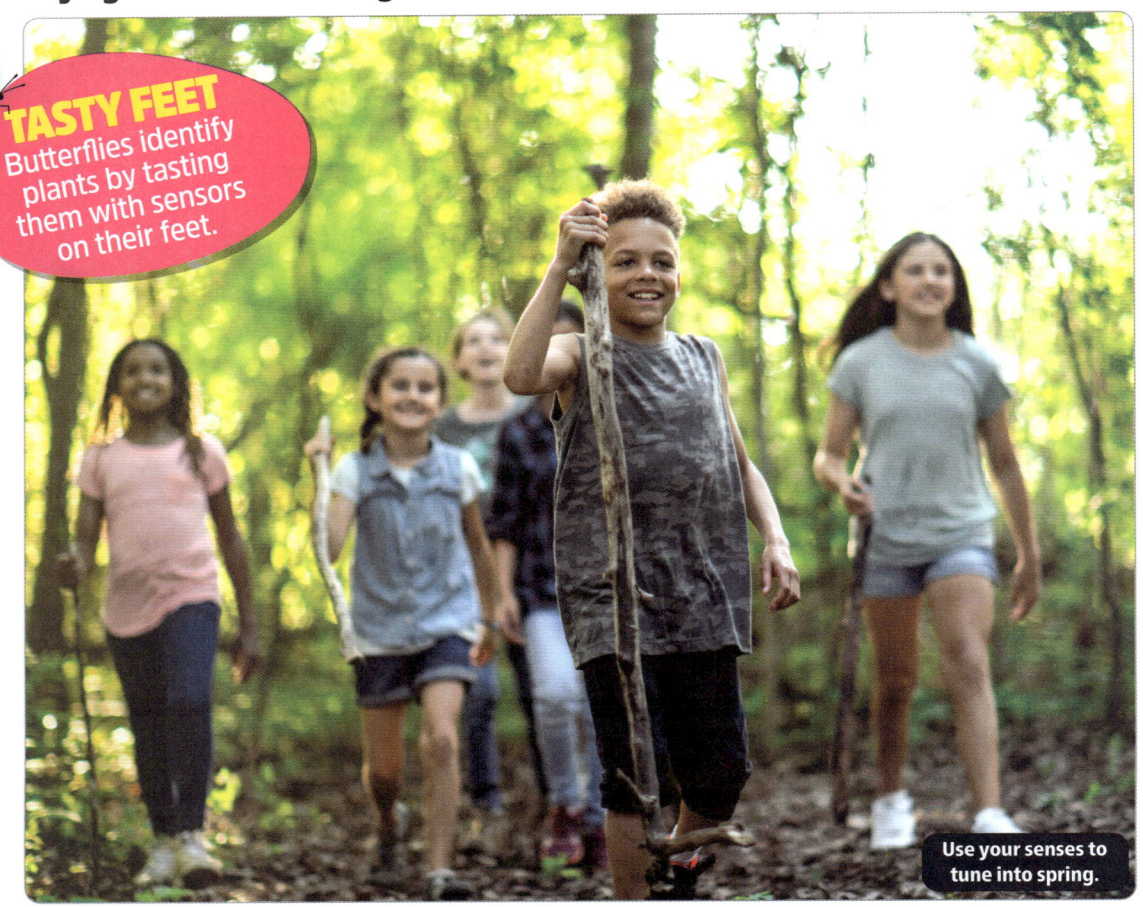

TASTY FEET
Butterflies identify plants by tasting them with sensors on their feet.

Use your senses to tune into spring.

Bring nature indoors

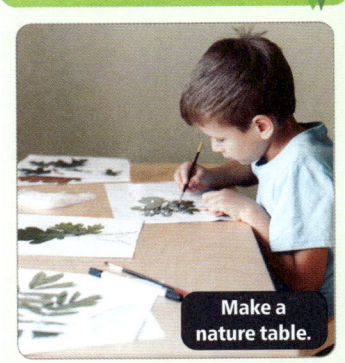

Make a nature table.

The Scottish Wildlife Trust suggests making a nature table. Collect sticks, feathers, fallen petals, leaves (nothing living) and whatever else you find interesting. Display them on a piece of paper on a table, shelf or windowsill. Write on the paper to identify or explain your finds. Take photos or show friends and family your nature display, noticing how the items change over time. When you're finished, try to return the items to where you found them.

Nature spotting

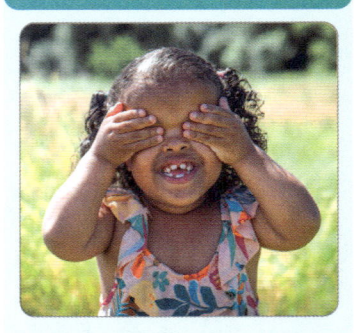

"I like spring because you can go out, as it is not too hot and not too cold. If it's windy you can go bird spotting and tick the boxes when you see each type of bird on your list. Birds and animals emerge from hibernation and we can hear them singing, chirping, and making noises. In spring, I like playing with my friends at the park. This spring I want to learn to ride my bike."
Mariama, aged eight

After months of winter, it lifts your spirits to see the natural world wake up in spring. You can enjoy spring the most by spending lots of time outside.

Look all around you
In springtime you can spot buds growing on trees and hedges, and flowers like daffodils, tulips and crocuses are blooming. Looking around your local area you might notice bees, butterflies, baby birds in a nest (never disturb a bird's nest), ducklings on a pond or river, or perhaps lambs in a field. Even in a city you can hear birdsong, find spider webs and see plants growing in pavement cracks. There are signs of spring all around if you look out for them.

Look up and enjoy nature's pleasures
When you're walking to school or a friend's house you can stop noticing what's around you because you're lost in thought – thinking about school, what you're going to eat for lunch or something that just happened. Mindfulness teacher Frances Trussell says being in the fresh air is a great way to focus on the present. "Your thoughts often take you on journeys into the past or future but by paying attention to what is here now you can enjoy life's little pleasures more and worry less. Looking up is an important thing you can do to help keep perspective – when you're next outside, look up and see if you can spot something that makes you feel uplifted."

Spot buds growing.

Use all your senses
You have several senses – sight, hearing, smell, taste and touch. Explore how many you can tune into when you're in nature. Can you feel the breeze or sun on your skin? Can you hear birds tweeting or leaves rustling? What else can you see or smell? Saying what you're noticing to yourself – out loud or just in your head – helps to keep your attention on the present moment instead of being distracted by other thoughts. If you're with a friend or family member, talk about what you're spotting. It will help you both enjoy your time outdoors. Taking photos of what you see can be an unwelcome distraction as you focus on taking the picture, so try taking a mental snapshot instead.

64

Enjoy the great outdoors

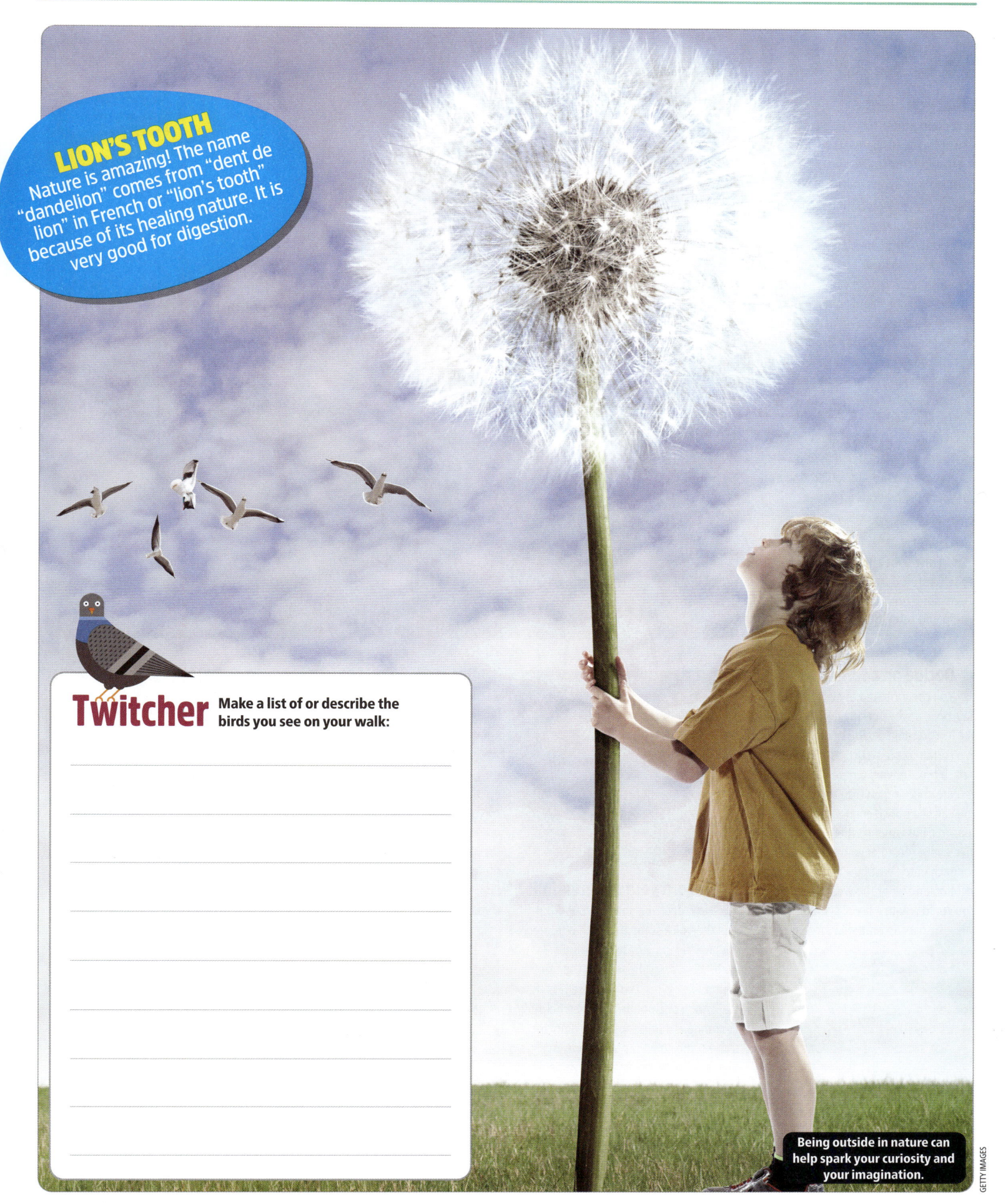

LION'S TOOTH
Nature is amazing! The name "dandelion" comes from "dent de lion" in French or "lion's tooth" because of its healing nature. It is very good for digestion.

Twitcher Make a list of or describe the birds you see on your walk:

Being outside in nature can help spark your curiosity and your imagination.

Mental wellbeing

Keep a nature diary

What you need
- A plain paper notebook (A4 is best)
- Drawing materials: pencils, crayons, paint

Do you love appreciating the natural world around you? Perhaps you notice colourful flowers on your walk to school or you have a favourite tree in your street. A nature diary is, quite simply, a way of recording the nature you come across. It's a great way to boost your observation skills and practise drawing and writing. You might also find it helps you to slow down and be more present in the moment.

Use your senses – sight, smell, touch (but check with an adult before you touch any plants) and hearing – to observe what's around you, and then put your observations on paper.

TOP TIP
Sit in one spot and notice what you hear and smell. Close your eyes for a few seconds – it will help you tune into your senses.

EPIC READ
Robert Shields is believed to have written the world's longest diary, at 35 million words.

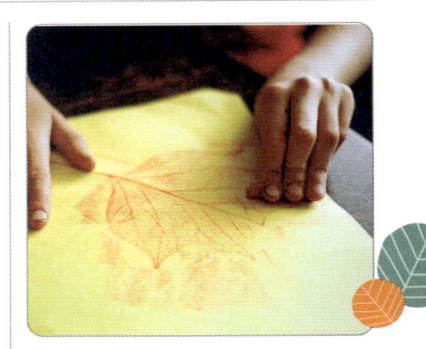

Keeping a nature diary is relaxing.

1 Decide on a format
You can write a diary entry every day, once a week or any time you feel like it. You could decide to record what's in a certain place – such as a local park – each time, or vary where you go. If you are checking on the same place you can see how it changes over the seasons, but varying where you go will give a nice record of your adventures. For each entry, write the date, time and location and what the weather is like. You could create a list of symbols for this – such as an umbrella for rain.

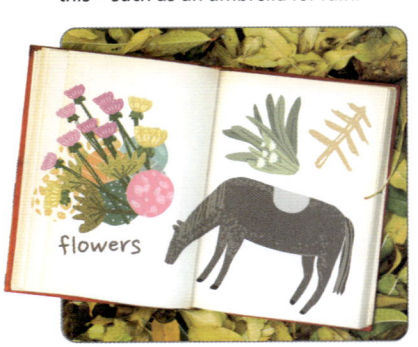

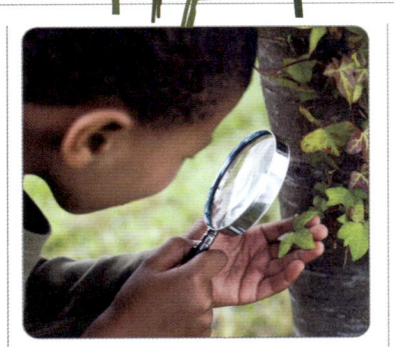

2 Record your observations
First, describe your surroundings and then pick some things that interest you, like an unusual leaf or a spider's web. What does the wind in the trees sound like? What can you smell? Is that stalk fuzzy or smooth? It can be helpful to compare things – perhaps a flower is the same colour as a postbox, or a beetle is the same size as a five pence coin. You can also write about how it makes you feel, what you think about it, or any questions you have. You could even compose a poem or a story.

3 Draw what you see
You can include a picture of a flowerbed, a single leaf or both. If you know the species of plant or creature you are drawing, write it next to the picture. You can always look it up later in a book or online. Putting measurements next to drawings is a useful way of keeping track of things as they grow. It might be easier to sketch things quickly in pencil and finish them later with paints or colouring pencils. If you have a camera, take pictures to help you remember colours and shapes.

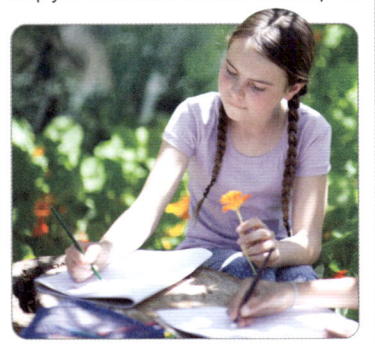

4 Take leaf or tree rubbings
This is a great way to record the wonderful patterns that occur in nature. To do a leaf rubbing you'll need a flat surface. Pick one if you have permission. Put the leaf under the page or some paper (you can cut it out and stick it in after). Use one hand to hold the paper firm and then take a plain or coloured pencil (the side, not the point) or a crayon, and gently rub it all over the leaf. An image of the leaf will appear on the paper. You can also do the same against the bark of a tree.

Head to theweekjunior.co.uk/activityhub for more crafts and recipes.

Keep a nature diary

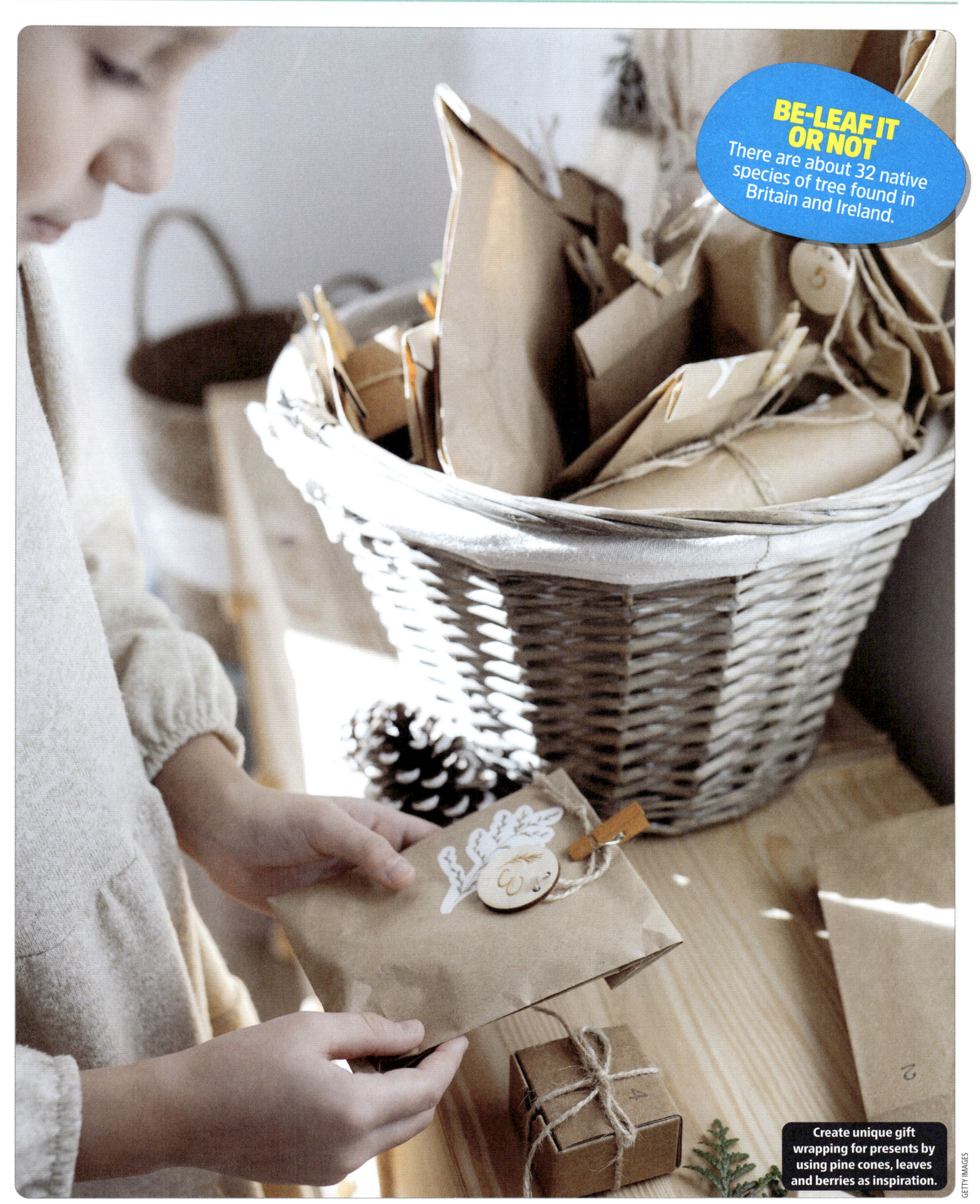

BE-LEAF IT OR NOT
There are about 32 native species of tree found in Britain and Ireland.

Create unique gift wrapping for presents by using pine cones, leaves and berries as inspiration.

Mental wellbeing

Get lost in music

Listening closely to different songs can boost your wellbeing.

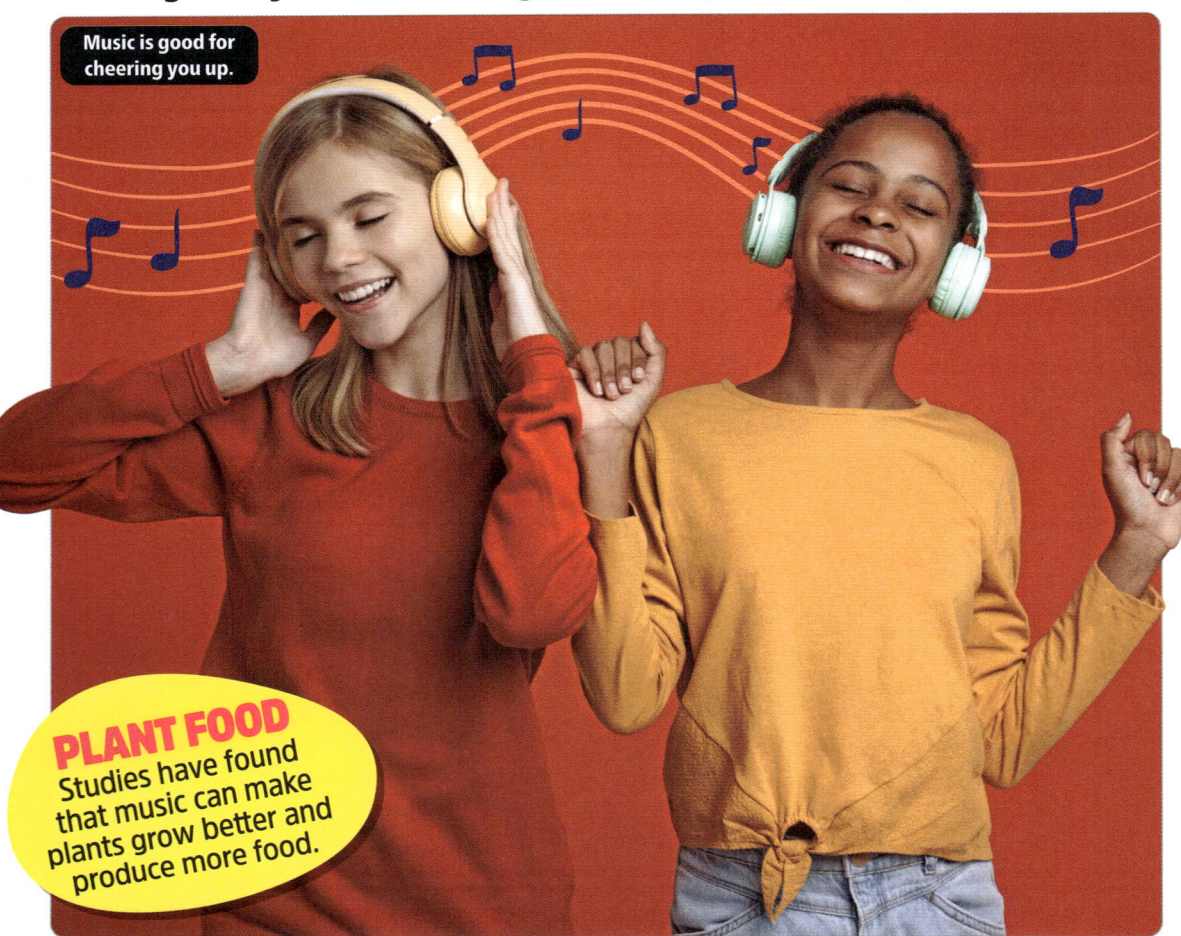

Music is good for cheering you up.

PLANT FOOD
Studies have found that music can make plants grow better and produce more food.

Have you noticed how upbeat, happy songs can give you energy, while calm, soothing tunes can help you unwind? Music really shapes people's moods, and getting lost in it can help you enjoy the magic of music even more.

What is "getting lost in music"?
This means concentrating on the music so hard you shut out your other thoughts for a short time. People often play tunes while they are doing something else, like reading a book or talking to friends. However, experts say if you try out different styles of music and listen closely to things like rhythm (the pattern of sounds), you boost its benefits and let it change how you are feeling in that moment.

How is it good for you?
Music is a language everyone understands and has brought humans together for thousands of years. Scientists say this is because it releases different chemicals in the brain that make you feel happy and closer to others. If you've studied for a test by singing your times tables you'll know how music can boost your memory. Research shows that listening to calm tunes reduces stress and even helps people feel less pain. In fact, music lights up nearly every part of the brain, says psychologist Jill Suttie (an expert in thoughts and feelings), and there could even be benefits that haven't been discovered yet.

Carnival dancers in Rio, Brazil.

How can you get lost in music?
Start by listening to types of music you haven't tried before, says author Ben Ratliff. Focus on different parts of the tune, such as rhythm. Listen to the drums and notice whether the pattern of beats stays the same or surprises you. Music from Cuba or Brazil, such as samba, is good for trying this. Listening while moving connects you closely to the sound, says Ratliff, so dance around your room and notice how the song changes. Use your senses to understand what the musician is trying to tell you, so imagine you can see, feel and even taste the song. Is it hard like metal or does it taste like melted chocolate? By listening carefully you can get the most from music – and have fun dancing too.

Music and you

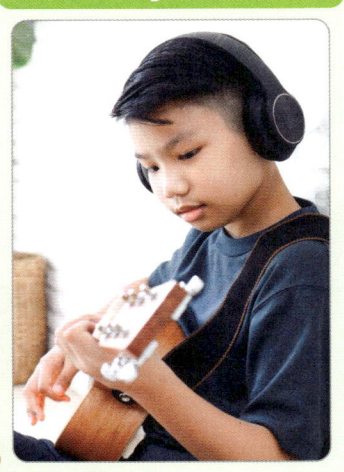

Think about your favourite song or track and ask:
- How does it make me feel?
- Why does it make me feel this way?
- Is the person who wrote the song trying to give me these emotions?

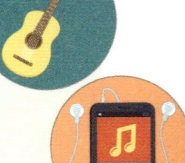

The different elements that go into a song

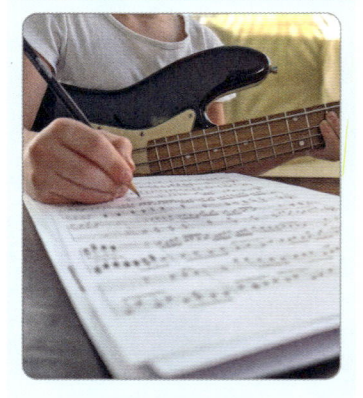

- **LYRICS** are the words.
- **MELODY** is the tune. It's the part of music you find yourself humming along to.
- **RHYTHM** is a pattern of sounds and silences throughout the song or track.

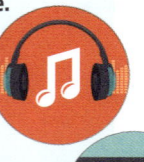

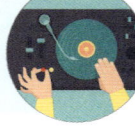

Get lost in music

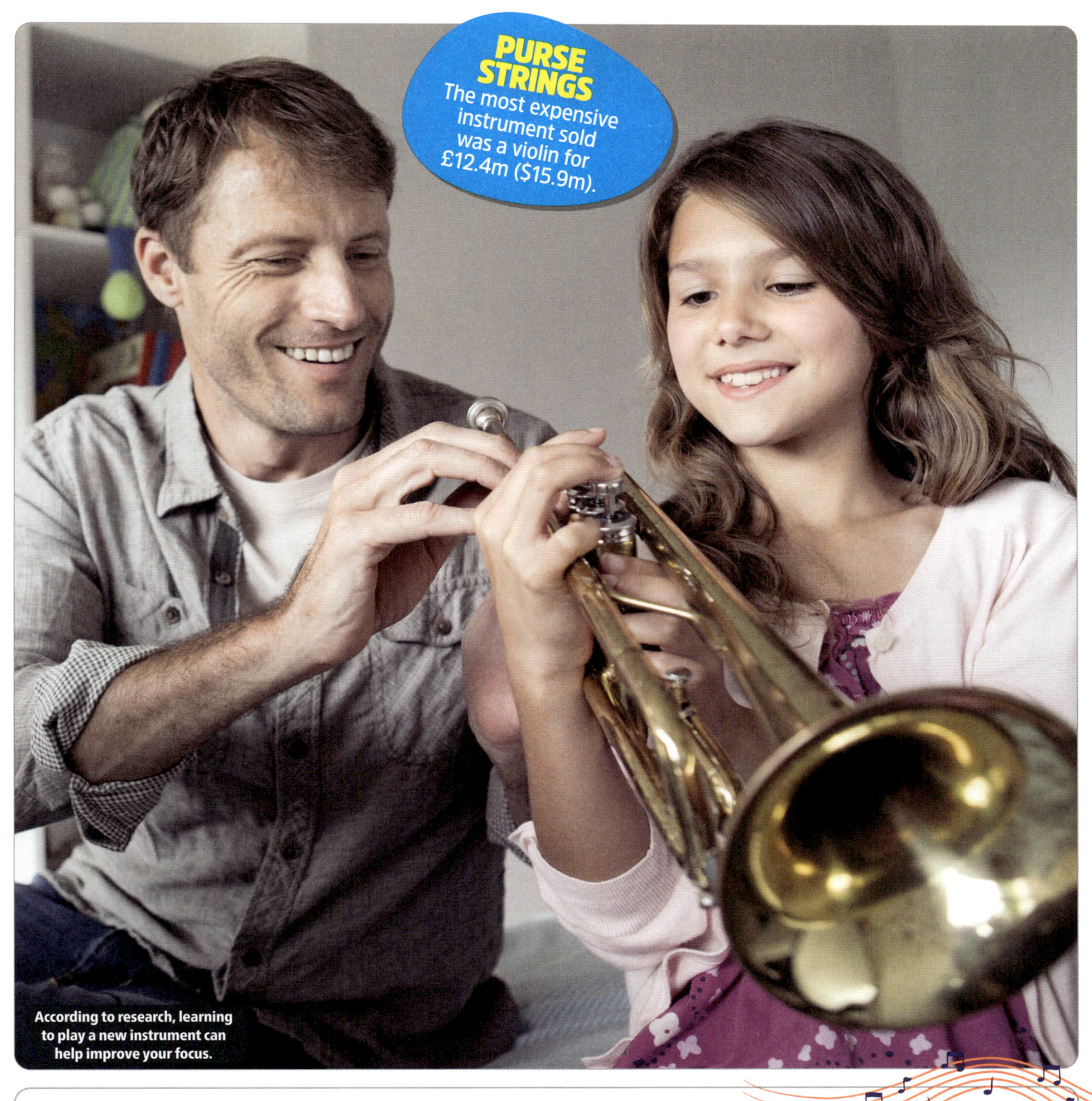

PURSE STRINGS
The most expensive instrument sold was a violin for £12.4m ($15.9m).

According to research, learning to play a new instrument can help improve your focus.

Make a playlist of all the songs that make you happy:

Mental wellbeing
Try journalling
Writing down your thoughts and feelings can boost your mental health.

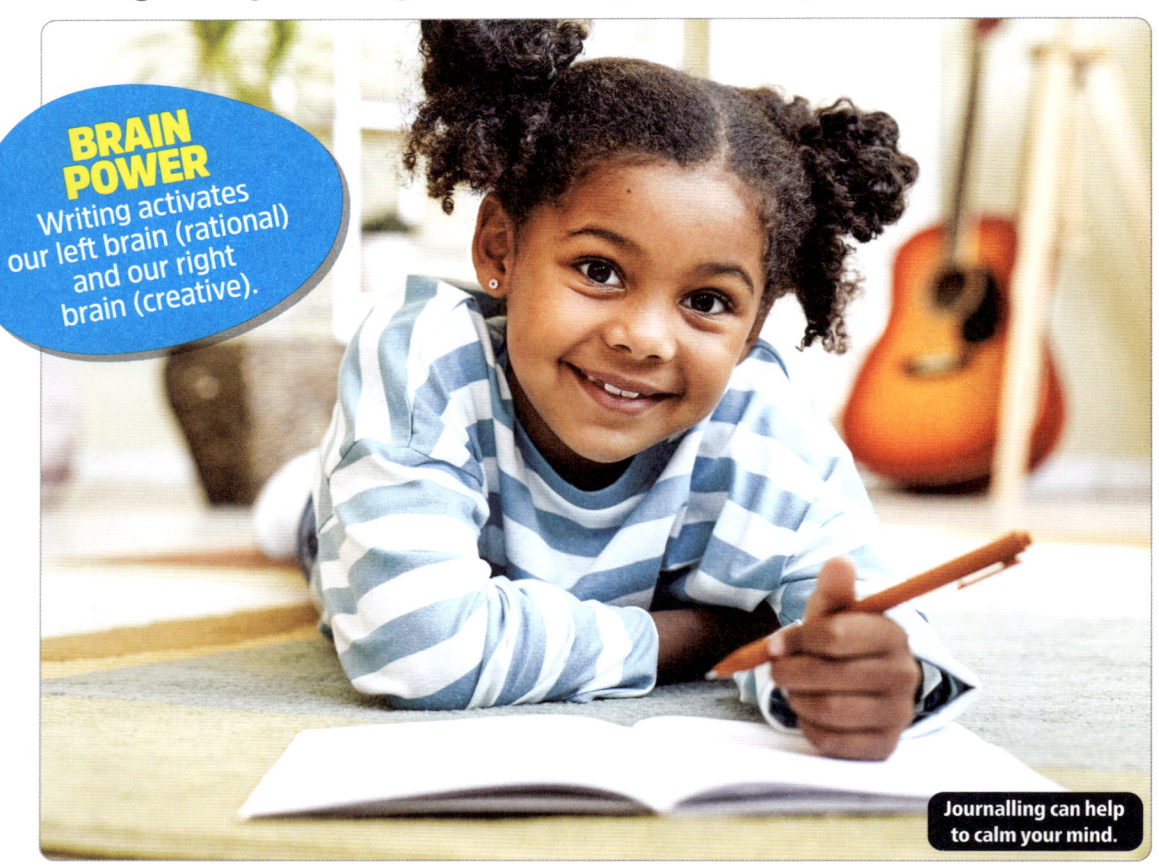

BRAIN POWER
Writing activates our left brain (rational) and our right brain (creative).

Journalling can help to calm your mind.

A diary is for keeping note of your day-to-day activities; a journal is where you can explore your thoughts.

What is journalling?
Journalling is writing down whatever you're thinking and feeling. It can include your dreams, fears, hopes, ideas and worries. You can use any notebook, it doesn't have to be a special one. Your journal is a place where you can write down what you find difficult to say out loud. You can use prompts or questions to guide your writing, such as, "What am I proud of?" or, "How can I be kind today?" (see panel for more suggestions), or you can write whatever comes into your mind. You don't have to keep what you've written. You can tear up the piece of paper afterwards if you like.

How journalling helps
Your journal is just for you. No-one else needs to see it, so you are free to write whatever you like. By writing in your journal you can work through a problem or puzzle as if you're in conversation with yourself.

Explore your feelings.

Chartered psychologist (an expert in thoughts and feelings) Suzy Reading advises doing a "brain dump" before bed. "Jot down all the things buzzing about in your head to calm your busy mind," she says. Cross off the things that you have no control over, or the things that don't actually bother you. "Highlight what you need to remember or work through, reminding yourself it's not time for that now, it's time to rest."

How to start journalling
You can start journalling straight away, all you need is paper and pen or pencil. If you want to be able to re-read your writing, choose a notebook to be your journal. Do you want to write when you feel like it or would you like to make it a habit? For example, you could write every day when you get home from school to help calm your mind. You can choose how long you write for or how much you write. Some days you might have more to say than on others. It isn't schoolwork so don't worry about spelling, grammar or punctuation. If you get stuck, Suzy Reading suggests drawing. "Even colours can be a helpful way to express yourself and let go. Don't pressure yourself to make it beautiful, this is about having fun and being yourself."

"I write and draw"

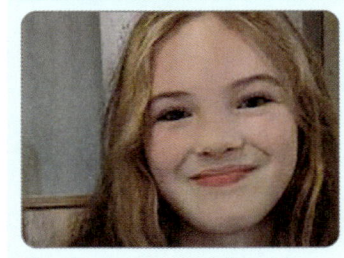

"I write in my journal and I draw as well. It's a *Harry Potter* one that is black leather and doesn't have lines. I don't do it every day but it is something I like to do. I have a *Wreck This Journal* as well and it is really good because every page tells you to do something to it, like throw it out of the window or scribble really hard."
Freya, aged 11

Ideas for your journal

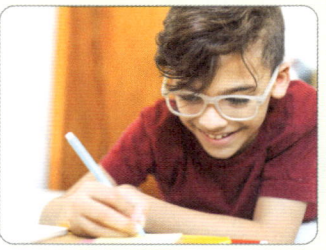

Try answering these journalling prompts from chartered psychologist Suzy Reading:

- What would I like to remember about today?
- What did I learn about myself or the world today?
- What went well today and why did that thing happen?
- What matters to me?
- What do I need today?
- What's on my mind today?
- What do I hope for in the future?
- Who is special to me and why?
- What made me laugh today?

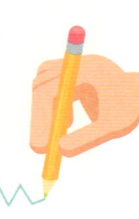

Try journalling

DAILY JOURNAL

Date:

Three things I'm grateful for today:

Today's rating: ★★★★★

What I did today:

Today I felt: ☹ ☹ 😐 🙂 😃

Because:

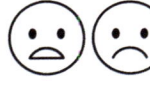

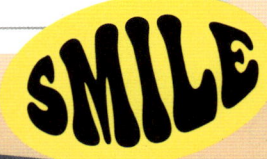

Mental wellbeing

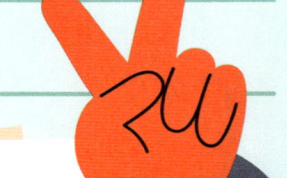

DAILY JOURNAL

Date:

Three things I'm grateful for today:

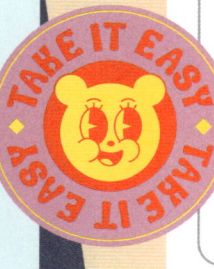

Today's rating: ★★★★★

What I did today:

Today I felt: ☹ ☹ 😐 🙂 😀

Because:

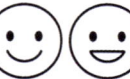

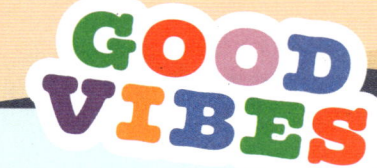

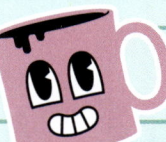

Try journalling

DAILY JOURNAL

Date:

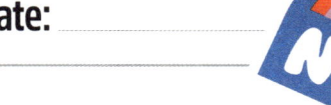

Three things I'm grateful for today:

Today's rating: ★★★★★

What I did today:

Today I felt: 😞 😟 😐 🙂 😃

Because:

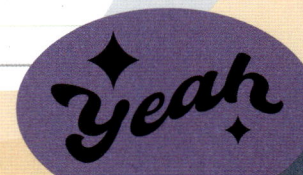

Mental wellbeing

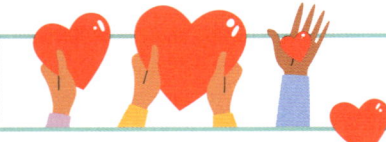

Love your mates

Friendships are important, so show your pals how much you value them.

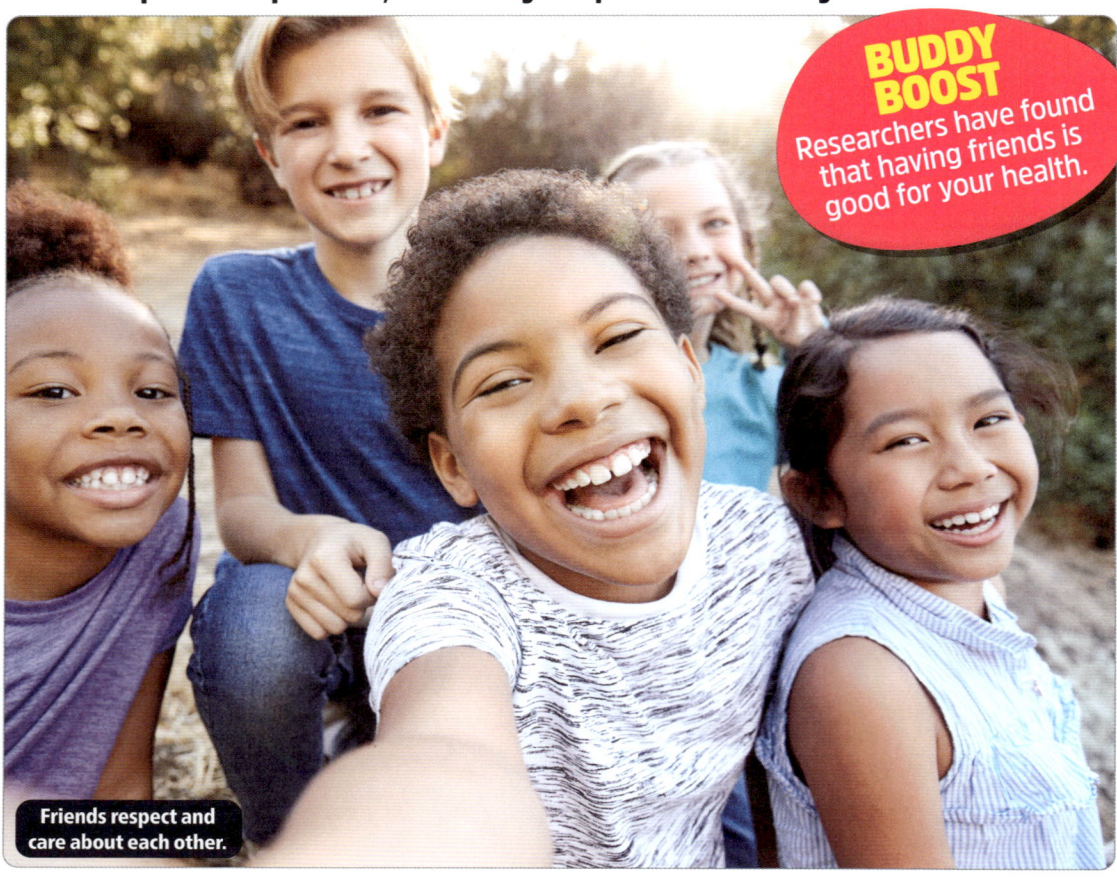

BUDDY BOOST
Researchers have found that having friends is good for your health.

Friends respect and care about each other.

Seven ways to make your friend feel fab

- Make them a card or present for their birthday.
- Share your snacks at break or lunch with them.
- Celebrate their achievements or when they've overcome a challenge.
- Really listen when they're telling you how they feel.
- Tell them what you like and admire about them.
- Take an interest in their hobbies.
- Remind them of their strengths and abilities when they're feeling unsure.

"I love my best friend"

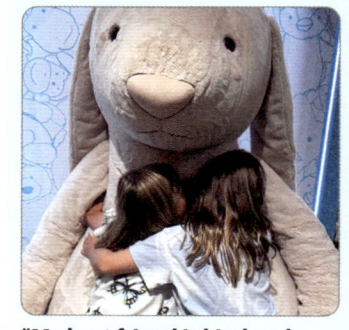

"My best friend is kind and caring. We love cuddly bunnies, gymnastics and playing together. We have lots of fun but when she's sad I try to make her feel better by giving her a big hug. We draw pictures and give them to each other and this makes her smile. When I'm sad my best friend tells me everything is going to be ok. I love my best friend."
Heidi, aged eight

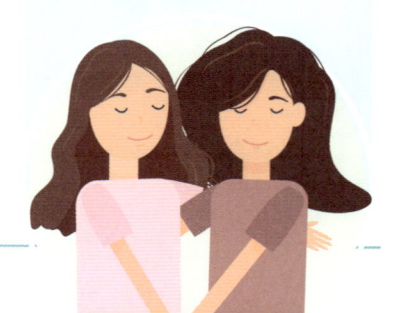

Whether you have one really good friend or hang out with several people, your mates are important.

Making friends
Your pals are the people you choose to spend time with. You might have friends at school, mates who live nearby or other people you hang out with at a club like Guides or football. You may see them every day or never meet in person if you connect with them online. It doesn't matter how many friends you have, what's important is that you and your friends respect and care about each other and enjoy spending time together. If a friend's behaviour is making you uncomfortable, young people's coach Maria Evans says it's ok to question it. "Being a supportive friend means you're willing to talk to them about behaviour you think is off. It might be tough but hearing it from you could have a positive impact on them."

Value your friendships
Evans says humans crave companionship. "Having a gang of friends and being part of a group not only makes you feel safe and seen, it's also really fun too. The world is full of exciting things to see and do, and sharing these experiences with a friend enriches them." One way to help your friend feel valued is to treat them as you would like to be treated. Think of what you would like someone who cares about you to do or say. How can you do the same for your friend?

Support your friends.

Be a good friend
Although you may be mates because you share common interests, like a favourite band or sport, your friends may be keen on different things too. Evans explains that you don't have to agree on everything. "It doesn't make that friendship any less special. Building a strong friendship means respecting and appreciating that your pal might have different opinions." A good friend encourages their mates to be themselves and loves them for who they are. Evans says, "Embracing differences creates a strong bond."
If a friend is having a tough time, let them know you're there to support them. That could be by encouraging or listening to them. Giving thought to the fun activities you do will make your pal feel valued and your time together more enjoyable. Plus, you will make treasured memories.

Love your mates

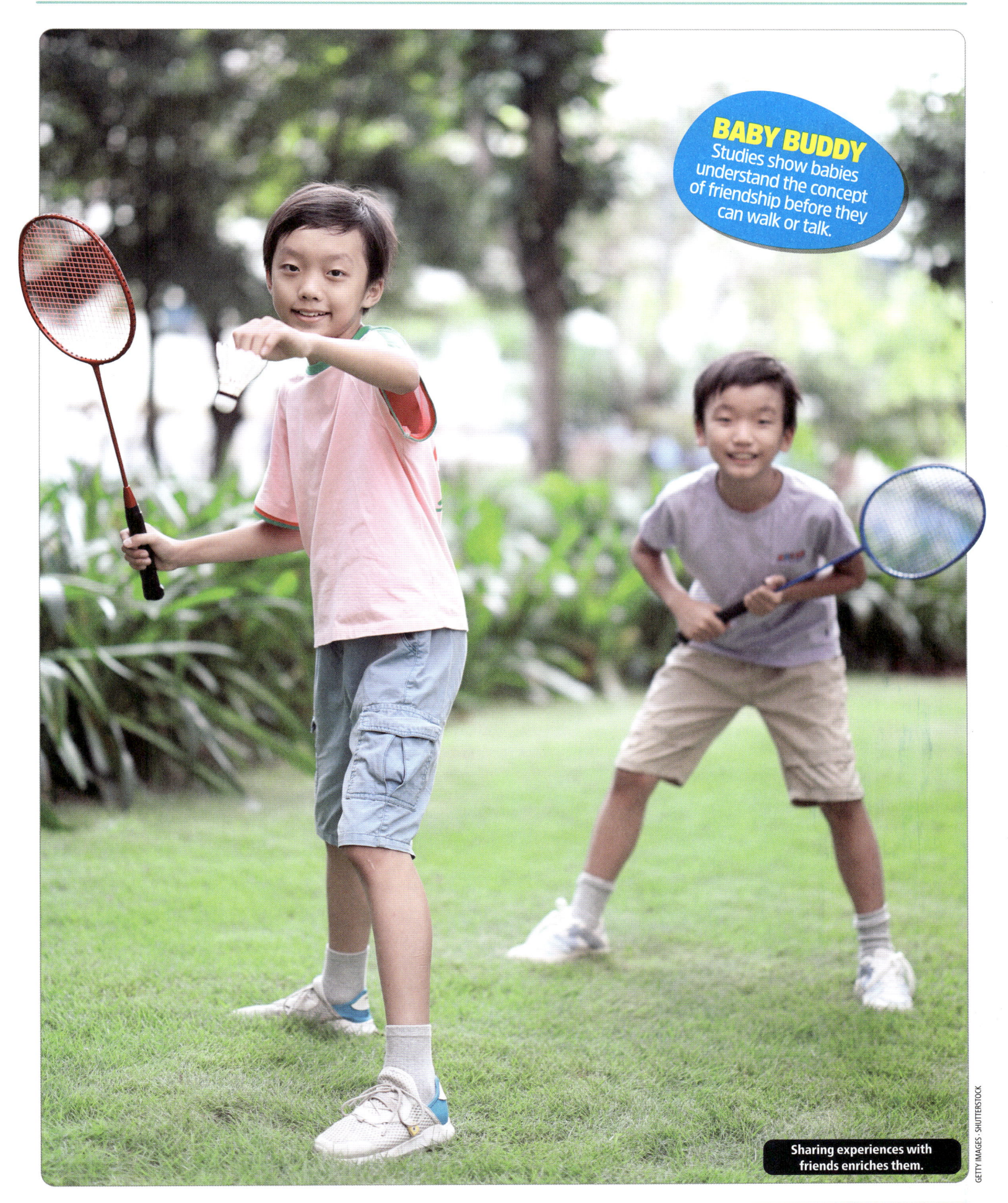

BABY BUDDY
Studies show babies understand the concept of friendship before they can walk or talk.

Sharing experiences with friends enriches them.

Mental wellbeing

The joy of joining in

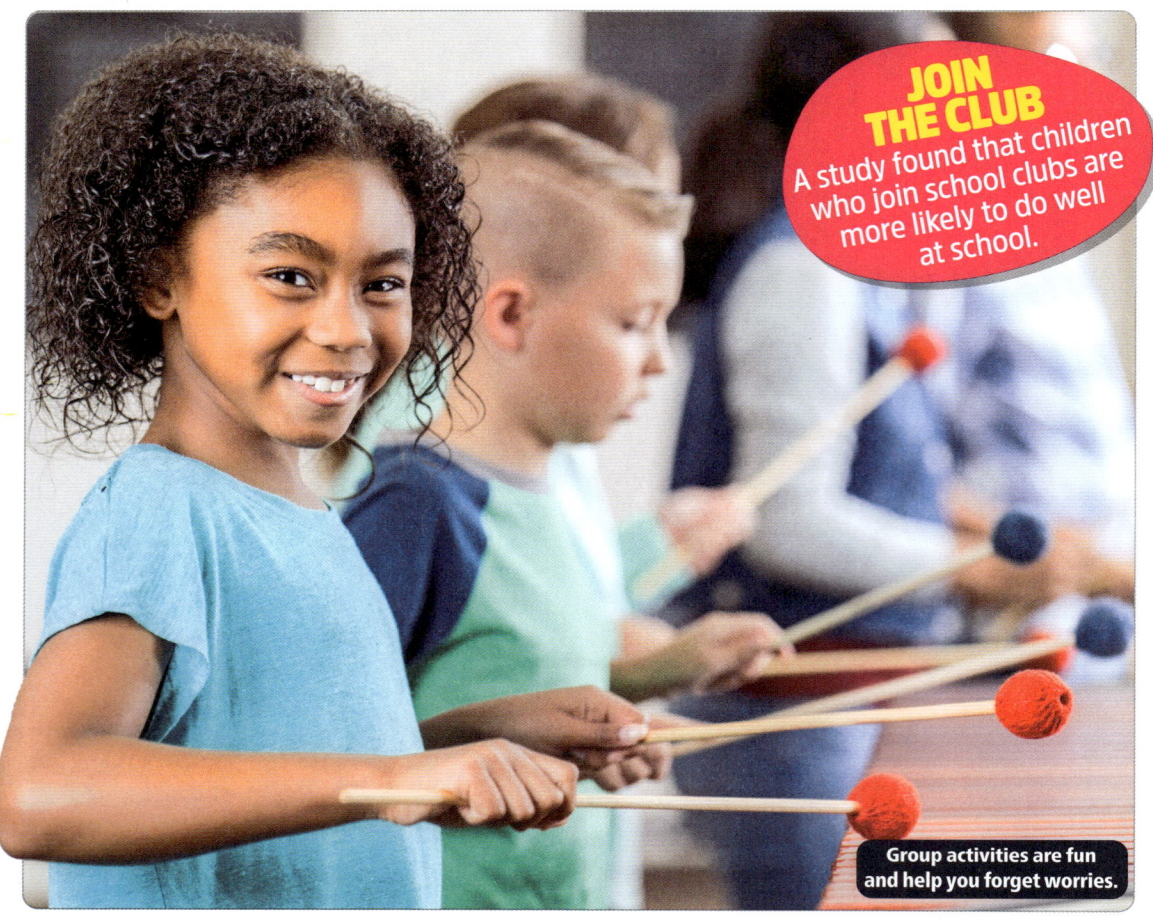

Getting involved in group activities is a great way to make new friends.

JOIN THE CLUB
A study found that children who join school clubs are more likely to do well at school.

Group activities are fun and help you forget worries.

Do you love feeling part of a group? Whatever your interests are, the new school year is a great time to join a club or activity, or even start your own.

Group activities build confidence
Whether you love music, sports, art or reading, there are lots of ways to join in group activities like a drama club or sports team. As well as meeting people who share the same interests as you, getting involved helps you discover skills you may not know you have. "Being part of a team can really give you confidence," says The Week Junior reader Jossie, aged 13. "Especially when you shout encouragement to each other or have a laugh about something that's happened. You also get to meet people who go to different schools or who are older than you, so it's a good way to make new friends."

What other benefits are there?
Joining in can be good for you in lots of ways. Working together involves teamwork. So in a music group, for example, everyone needs to practise their part and listen to how everybody else is playing. As well as improving your music skills, this strengthens communication and boosts your self-esteem (how you feel about yourself). Rochelle Eime, who studies the benefits of sport, says being part of a sports team involves overcoming challenges. "You've got to train and work hard; you learn to win and more importantly learn to lose," she explains, which can also help you deal with stress. Research has even found that feeling connected to others in clubs and groups can make us healthier and live longer.

Jossie enjoys being in a team.

How to get more involved
The new school year is a really good time to try something new. Even if you haven't liked a sport or a group activity before you may enjoy being part of the team now. "Give it a go," says Nikita Parris from England's football team. So ask at your school or local library about free clubs, or get together with friends and start your own. Whatever you do it's important to remember to laugh and have fun. "You're playing with your friends and you're making new relationships and friendships," says Parris.

Benefits of teamwork

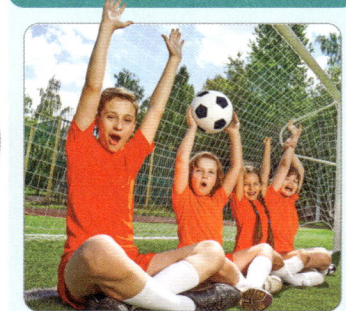

- **Stay motivated.** Being part of a team means relying on each other. This makes it easier to stick at a sport, even when you lose.
- **Make friends.** Spending lots of time together and building trust helps you connect with others.
- **Build confidence.** Learning new skills together and developing them can boost your confidence.

Top tips for starting your own club

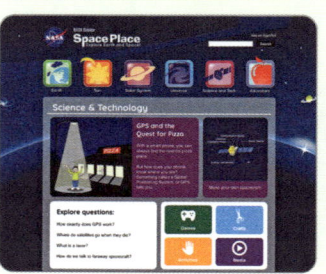

- **Astronomy or space club.** Find activity ideas and follow the latest space adventures here spaceplace.nasa.gov
- **Gardening club.** Learn how to sow seeds, care for plants and get some ideas at tinyurl.com/TWJ-gardenclub
- **Debating club.** Pick a topic to debate and make sure everyone gets a chance to speak. Find fun debating games here tinyurl.com/TWJ-DebatingClub

The joy of joining in

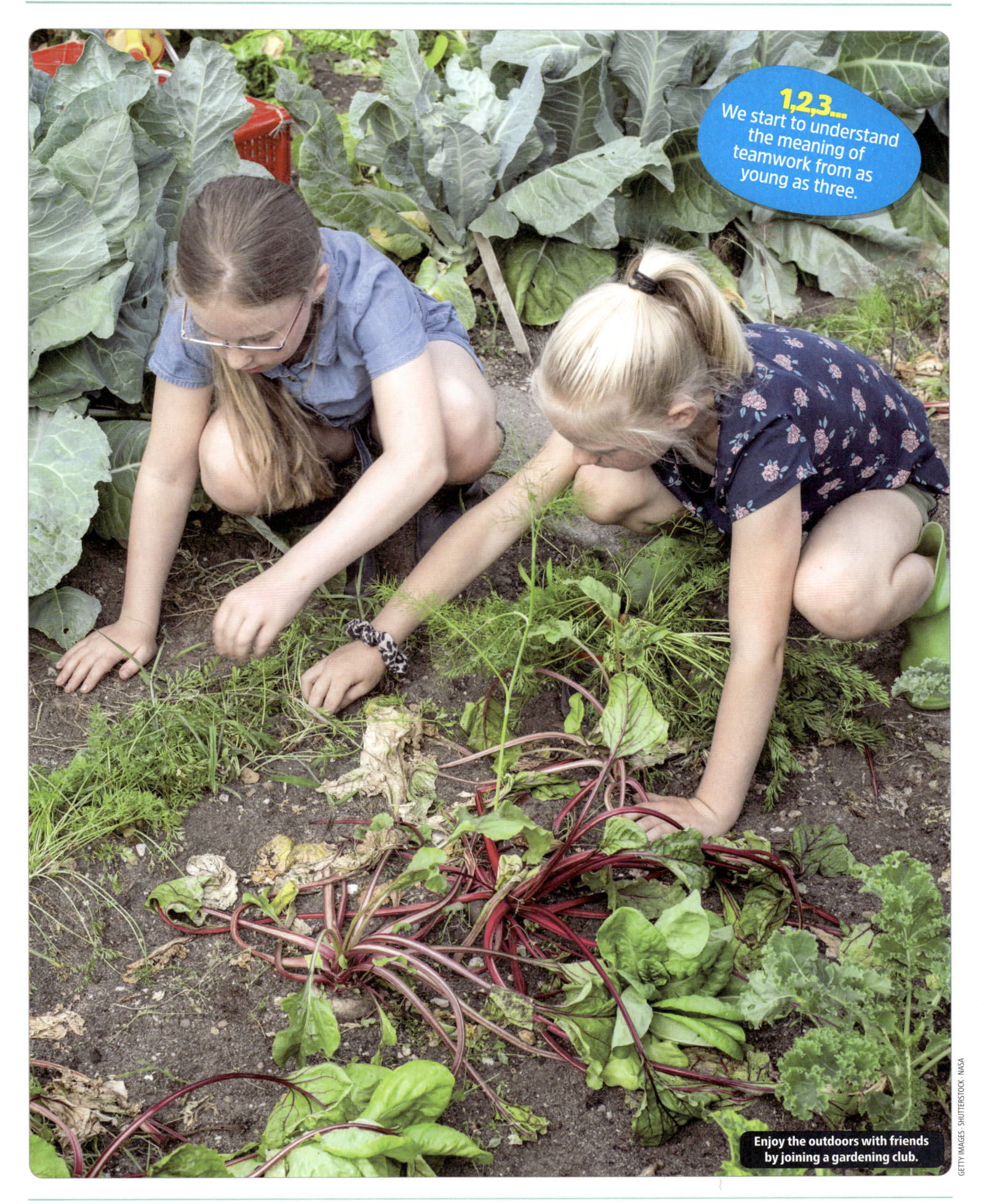

1,2,3... We start to understand the meaning of teamwork from as young as three.

Enjoy the outdoors with friends by joining a gardening club.

Mental wellbeing

Find your passion

Doing something you love helps you forget your worries.

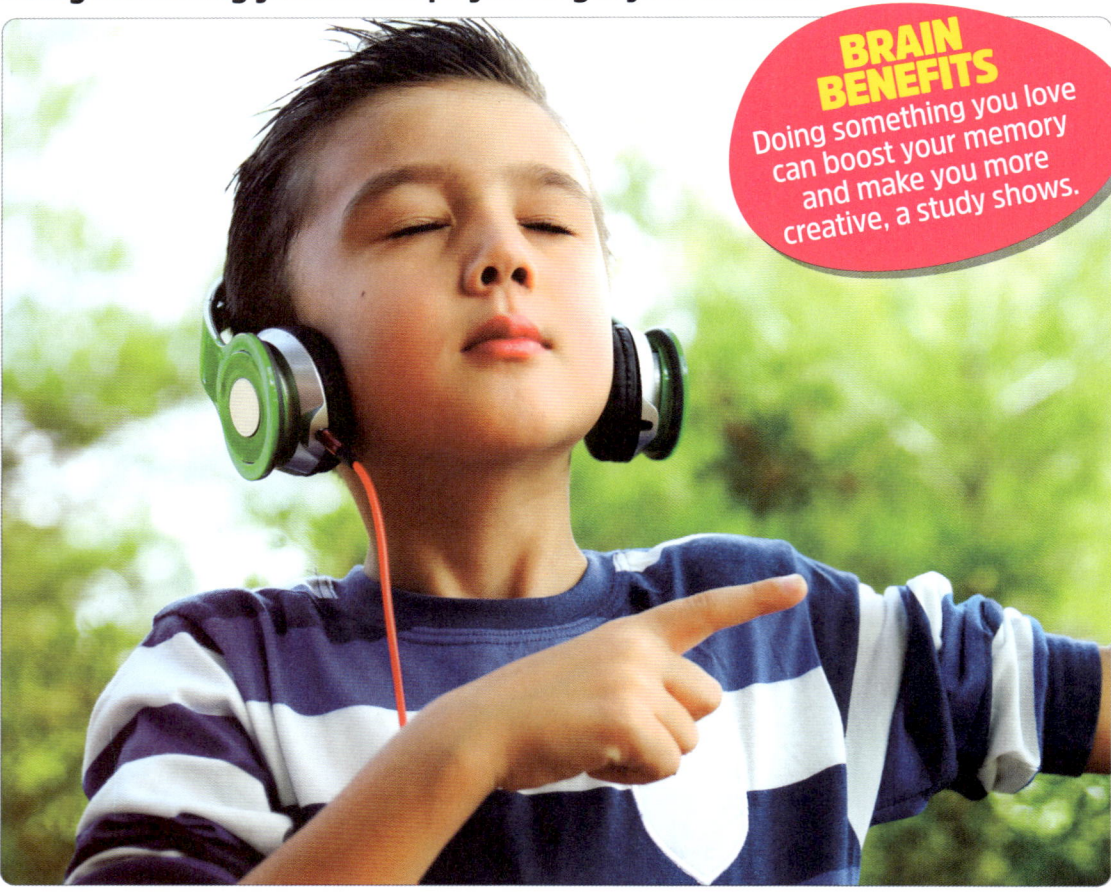

BRAIN BENEFITS
Doing something you love can boost your memory and make you more creative, a study shows.

Is there something you love doing more than anything else? Discovering you have a passion for a sport or hobby not only brings you joy – it can also boost your self-esteem (how you feel about yourself) and make you more confident.

What is a passion?
Passion describes the strong feeling you have when doing something you love. This could be anything from listening to music, playing sports, drawing, doing puzzles or getting lost in a book. Dr Alison Block, an expert in thoughts and feelings, says following your passion doesn't mean trying to be the best at something or doing it because other people want you to. What matters is you're drawn to an activity because of how it makes you feel. "It's something that touches your heart and mind," says Block.

Finding your flow
When you're doing something you're passionate about, you feel less stressed because you can forget your worries, Block explains. You can go into a "flow state", when your mind and body are completely absorbed by what you're doing. When this happens, difficult thoughts and feelings melt away and all that matters is what's in front of you. If your passion involves learning a new skill or sport then it can help you to discover your strengths. Block says this can build your self-esteem and also teaches you to overcome challenges while doing something you love.

Try new things to find what you love.

Discover your passion
Finding a passion makes it sound as if your ideal activity is sitting around, waiting to be discovered, says Paul O'Keefe, an expert in human behaviour. However, passion often begins with a spark of curiosity and grows from there. This spark could be lit by anything, like an inspiring lesson or an exciting goal in a football match. Following this spark can turn it into something meaningful that lifts your heart, O'Keefe says. Block recommends exploring different things. "You can discover a passion by trying new activities," she says. Then make time for it. Passion can also be catching, she says. So share interests with your friends and help them find their passion too.

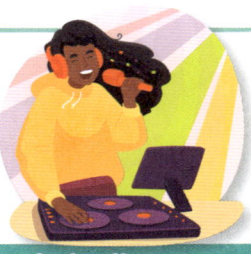

Tips to help discover your passions

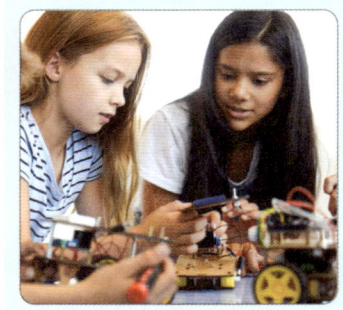

- **Try something new, like auditioning for the school play, doing a junior parkrun or visiting an art gallery.**

- **Write a list of things you enjoy, for example, camping, exploring woods and climbing trees. See if there's a thread that connects them, such as exploring the outdoors.**

- **Join a club to get inspired by other people who share your interests. Ask at school or your local library for ideas.**

Ask yourself

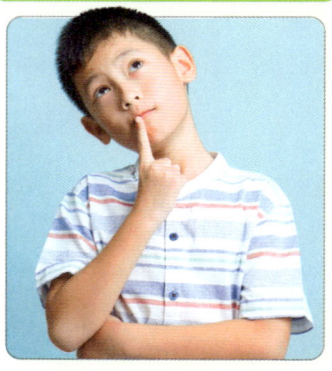

- **What are the things that I love to do?**
- **What gives me energy and excitement?**
- **Are there activities I always want to do and others that I put off?**
- **What can I talk about for ages that makes me smile?**

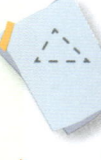

Find your passion

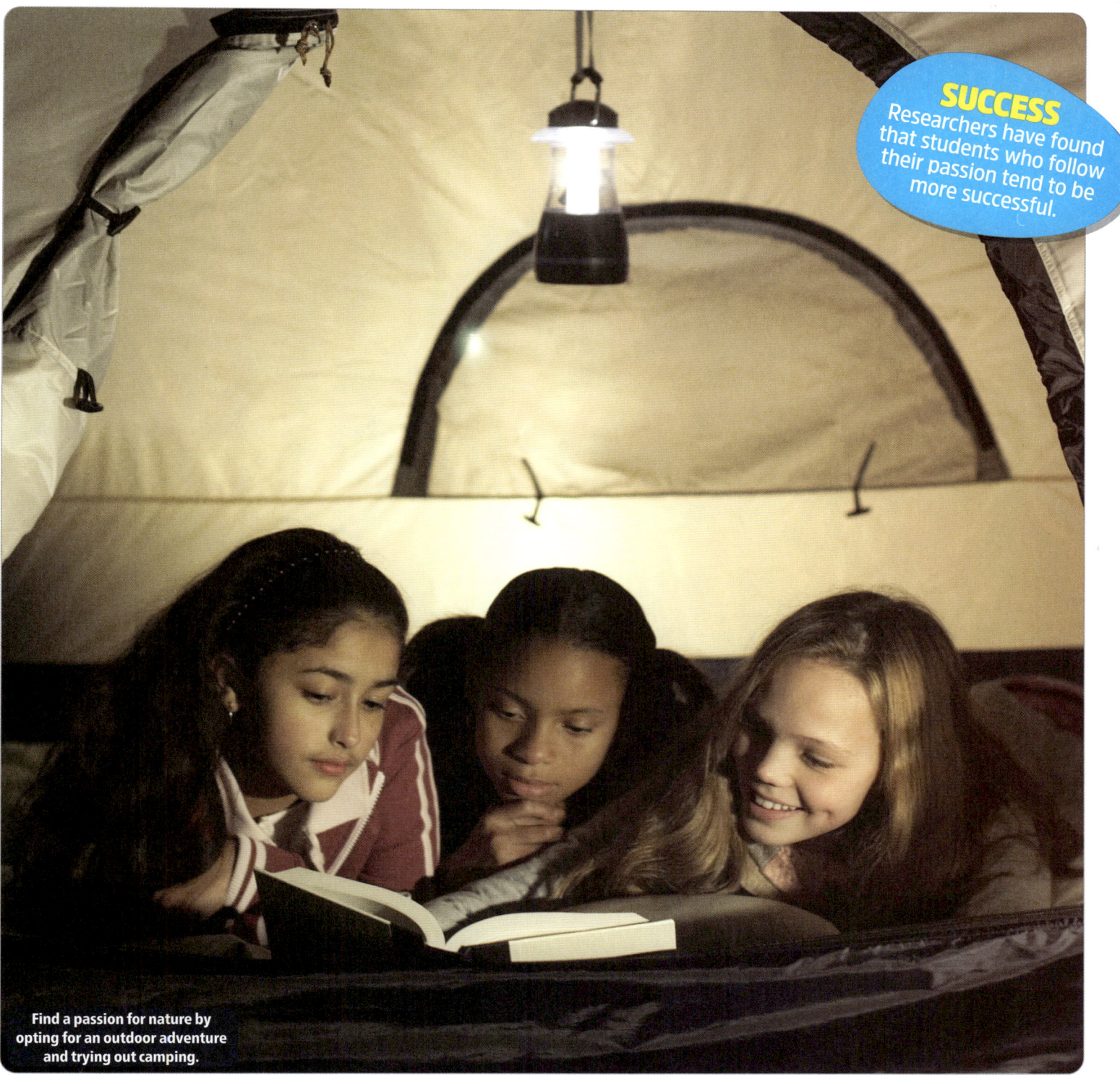

SUCCESS
Researchers have found that students who follow their passion tend to be more successful.

Find a passion for nature by opting for an outdoor adventure and trying out camping.

Make a list of things that you love to do:

Mental wellbeing

Make a difference
Do something to help others in your life.

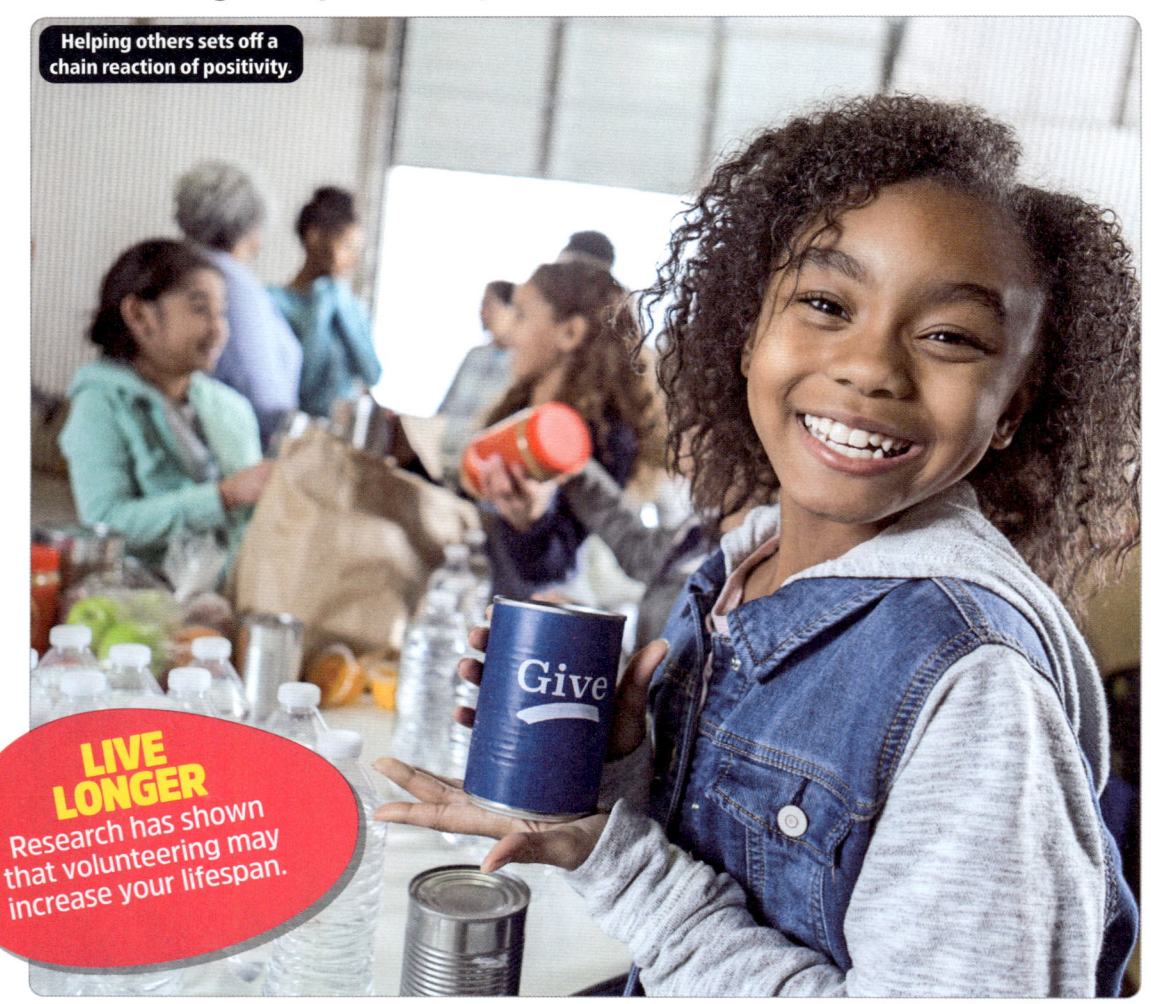

Helping others sets off a chain reaction of positivity.

LIVE LONGER
Research has shown that volunteering may increase your lifespan.

Making a difference to other people doesn't only do good for them – you can benefit too. Try to do something helpful in the local community. It doesn't need to be something big or that takes up a lot of time or costs any money. It's simply doing something to help make someone else's life a bit better.

How you can make a difference?
There are lots of ways you can make a difference to people close to you and those you might never meet. Helping out at home by laying the table for dinner or cleaning your room without being asked makes a difference. Being kind to someone in the playground or joining the school council helps you to make a difference at school. You can make a difference in your local community by giving your unwanted books, clothes or toys to charity or taking part in a litter pick. Young people's coach Maria Evans says that doing something meaningful for another person can set off a chain reaction of positivity. "Your actions show them they matter, which can boost their self-esteem. Trust and connection grow, making your relationship stronger. Your kindness might inspire them to help others too."

It makes you feel good
When you do something nice for someone else you're showing yourself that you can have a positive impact. It empowers you, you feel able to make a real difference – which is important when life can seem difficult at times. Volunteering is a great way to make a difference. You might think it's just about helping others but Evans says it's great for your wellbeing too. "It's a chance to meet new people, strengthen friendships and create memories. It's a brilliant way to boost your confidence because when you use your skills it reminds you that you matter and have the power to create change."

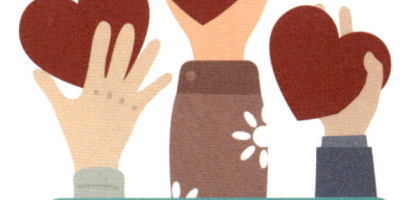

Can you help out at school?

How to be a great helper
You can make a difference to other people any day. Here are some ideas to try out:

- Help a classmate with schoolwork.
- Do a sponsored event to raise money for charity.
- Tell someone that you appreciate them.
- Help a neighbour by clearing litter on your street.
- Join in a beach clean.
- Make a card to say thank you to someone.
- Ask each member in your household what you could do that would make a difference to them.

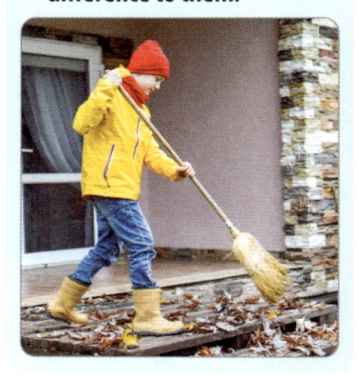

"I enjoy helping younger kids"
"Last year in primary school I helped out in a Year 1 class every week. I helped them with their work. I also read with them. I enjoy helping younger kids. And it benefitted them because it gave them some extra one-to-one support and helped to grow their confidence talking with older children in the school. I enjoyed working with them and supporting their learning journey at school."
Rapha, aged 11

80

Make a difference

Choose a charity and use this page to design a poster to raise awareness for the cause.

Mental wellbeing

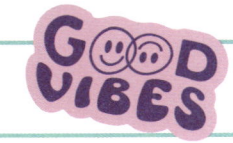

Make a noise about bullying

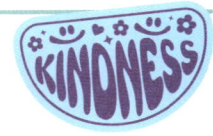

Speaking up and being kind to others is good for you too.

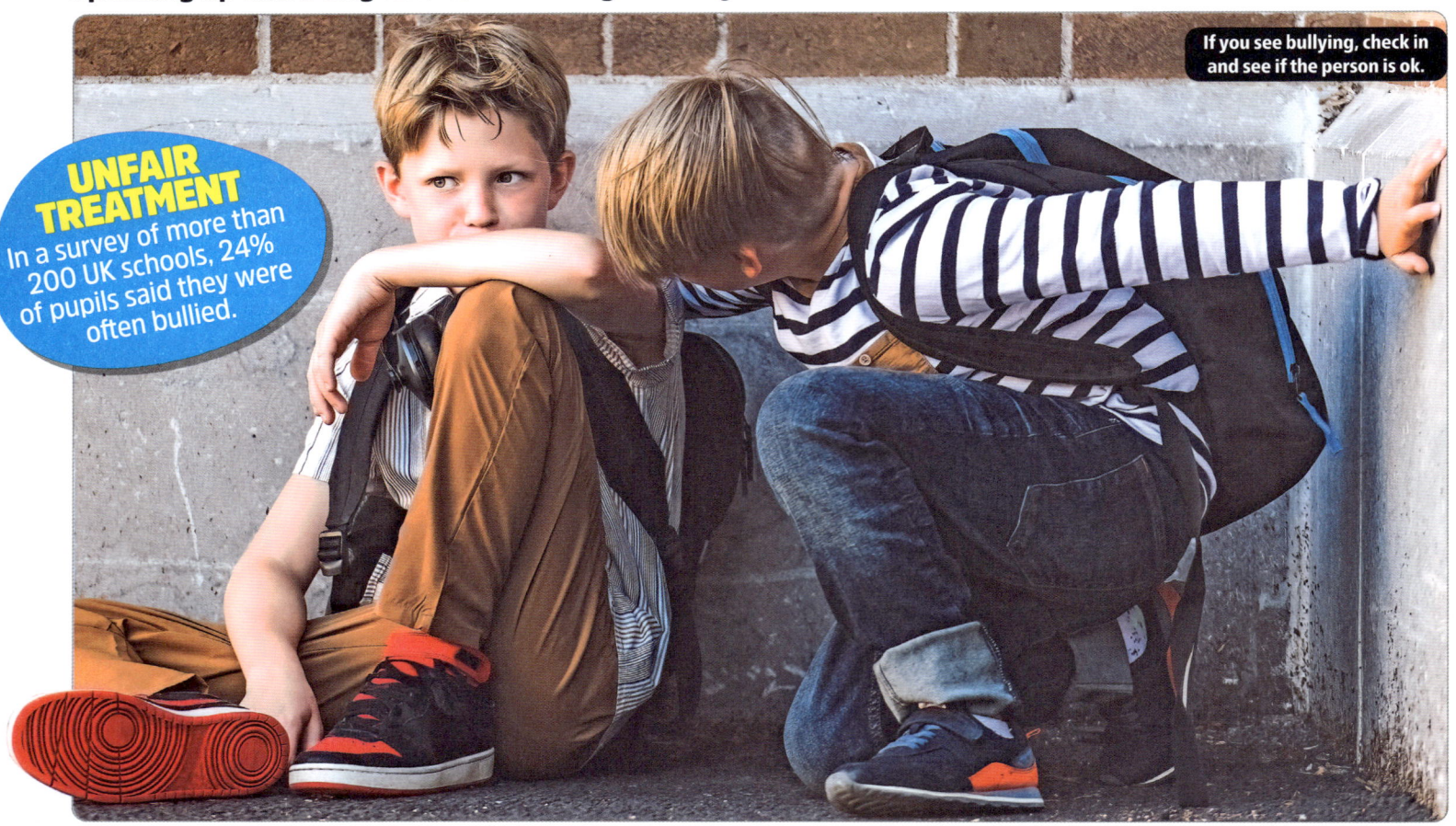

If you see bullying, check in and see if the person is ok.

UNFAIR TREATMENT
In a survey of more than 200 UK schools, 24% of pupils said they were often bullied.

Did you know that kindness has the power to change the world and everyone can help stop the hurt caused by bullying?

What is bullying?
Bullying is when one person or a group of people use their power to hurt someone else. The Anti-Bullying Alliance (ABA) says people can have power over others for lots of reasons. These may include being older, bigger or stronger; being able to communicate better; or being part of a group when the other person is on their own. Bullying involves using this power to hurt someone with words or actions, and it can happen face to face or online (called "cyberbullying"). Bullying is never acceptable, says the ABA, and it's important to know that it's never your fault if you're being bullied.

How can kindness help?
People have the power to hurt but they also have the power to be kind. Small acts can make a big difference, like asking someone at school who is sitting on their own to join your group or play in your game. Jaime Thurston set up the charity 52 Lives, which is a member of the ABA and runs kindness workshops in schools. She says, "Kindness can be seen as soft and fluffy, but it's so important to our wellbeing." Studies show that kindness reduces stress, boosts self-esteem (how you feel about yourself) and releases feel-good chemicals in your brain. So as well as helping others, you're being kind to yourself, too.

Talk to an adult if you're being bullied.

Make a noise about bullying
To help combat bullying we need to make a noise about it. Martha Evans from the ABA says, "If you see someone else being bullied you shouldn't silently accept it. Instead, ask the person if they're ok, call it out or let someone know what is happening." This may also include keeping a record of what happens and when. "This will be useful when you discuss it," she explains. If you're being bullied, don't be tempted to fight back, Evans says. "You might be hurt even further or be seen as the problem. Instead, walk away and seek help."

The difference between banter and bullying

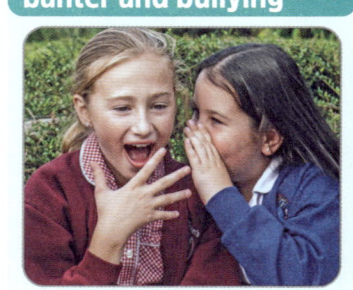

It can be difficult to tell the difference between "just a joke" or "banter", and bullying. If jokes are always made about the same person and target something personal like appearance, religion or how clever they are, this could be bullying. "Ask yourself, how would I feel if those comments were being made about me?" says Martha Evans. "If you'd be hurt or someone tells you it's hurting them, it's not banter."

POSITIVE ENERGY

Make a noise about bullying

Fill in the sheet below and talk about these areas with friends or family to get to grips with how to help someone being bullied.

Verbal ways to bully:

What might someone being bullied think?

Emotional ways to bully:

What might someone being bullied feel?

Mental wellbeing

My voice matters

Sharing your thoughts can ease your worries and help you feel calm.

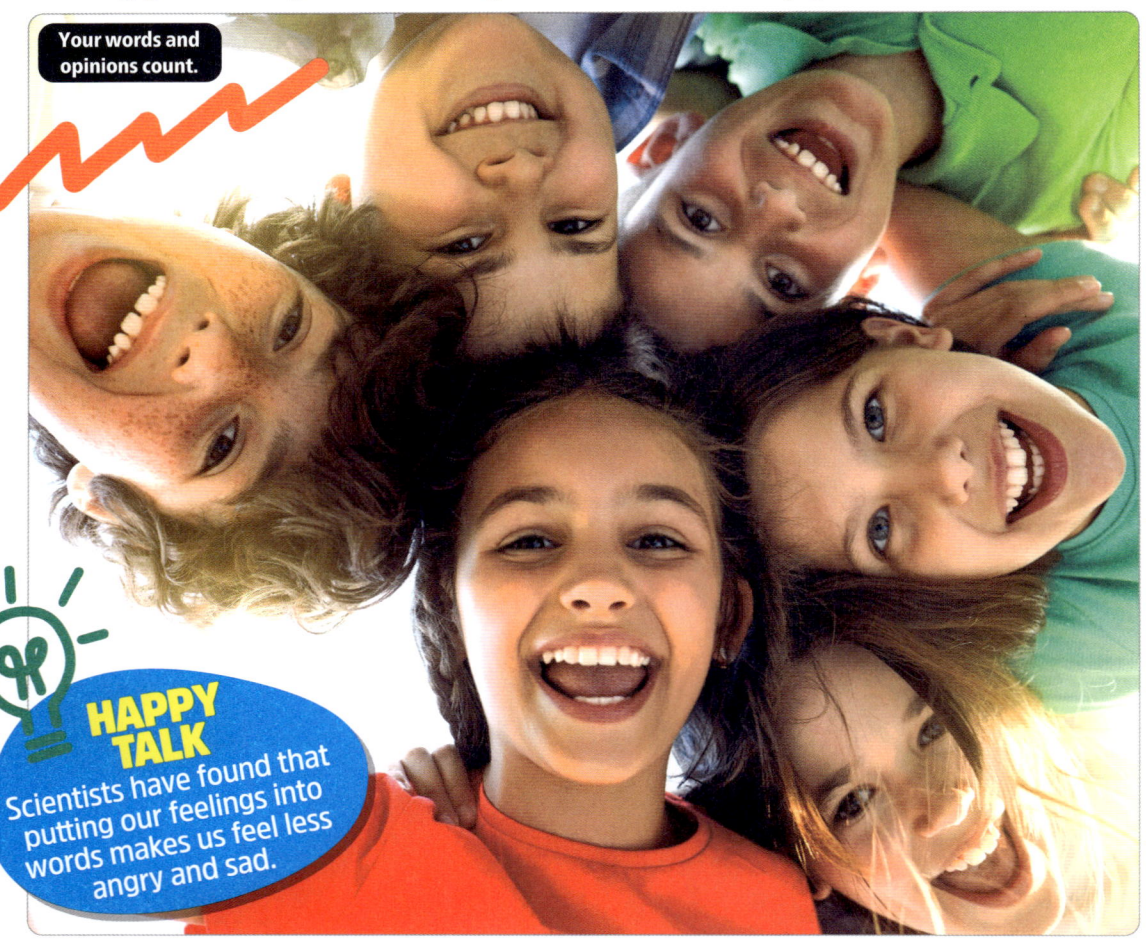

Your words and opinions count.

HAPPY TALK
Scientists have found that putting our feelings into words makes us feel less angry and sad.

Finding the words to explain how you feel isn't always easy. This is why it's important to speak up and make your voice heard.

What does speaking up mean?
Do you have trouble sharing your thoughts – or worry no one will listen if you do? Making your voice heard means understanding that your words matter and your opinions count. Dr Julia Clements is a psychologist (an expert in thoughts and feelings) at Place2Be. She tells *The Week Junior* it means "expressing your views, thoughts and feelings, not bottling them all up, and being open to hearing the thoughts, feelings and views of others too." Making yourself heard isn't about shouting the loudest; in fact you don't have to use your voice at all. You can express what you like and don't like or what you want for the future by writing or drawing instead, says Clements. "It's about finding ways to share what matters to you," she explains.

Practise with friends.

Why is it important?
Sharing your feelings with a person you trust will help you make sense of them. Scientists have discovered that sharing your feelings triggers a feel-good chemical in your brain that makes you feel relaxed and calm. Your voice can make a big difference to other people too, including friends and siblings. Jaime Thurston is from a charity called 52 Lives, which delivers kindness workshops in schools. She says, "You can spread kindness and happiness simply by speaking. With a few kind words, you could help someone feel good about themselves or let them know they are supported."

How can you find your voice?
Clements suggests practising conversations with friends, parents or carers. If you're struggling to explain your feelings, find a way that feels right for you, whether it's talking face-to-face or writing it down. When you're ready, "Take a deep breath and believe in yourself," says Thurston. "Know that your opinion matters."

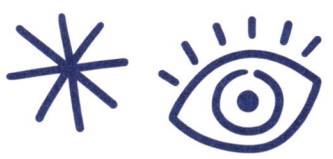

Children's rights
Your right to express your views, thoughts and feelings, and to have them taken seriously, is part of the United Nations Convention on the rights of the child. This is an agreement by the United Nations (an organisation of 193 countries that work together on climate change and peace) that adults and governments must work together to protect and improve children's rights.

Top tips to find your voice and be heard

- If you're confused about something, don't be afraid to ask questions.
- Do you find it difficult to express yourself with words? Try this fun art activity on the opposite page and "make a swirl" to share what matters to you.
- Write a letter to your MP or local newspaper to support something you believe in, like recycling or new facilities at your local park.
- Tell a trusted friend or adult about how you feel and what they can do to help.

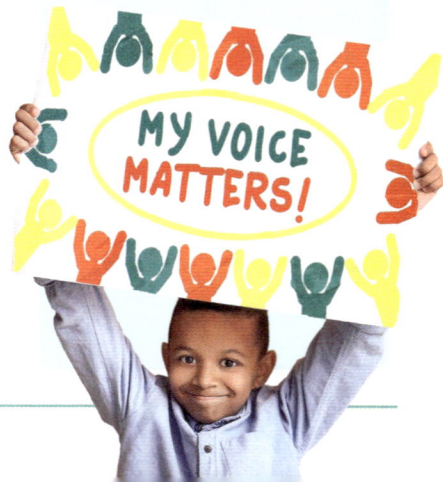

MY VOICE MATTERS!

Express yourself

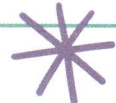

Express yourself

Create a colourful swirl to share what things matter to you the most.

This activity was created by charity Place2Be to help you express your personality. Just fill the swirl with words and pictures that highlight the things that matter to you.

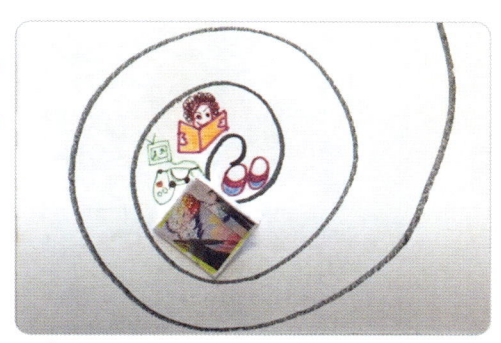

1. Start in the middle with day-to-day things – like your family, friends, toys and home. For example, a picture of your favourite book.

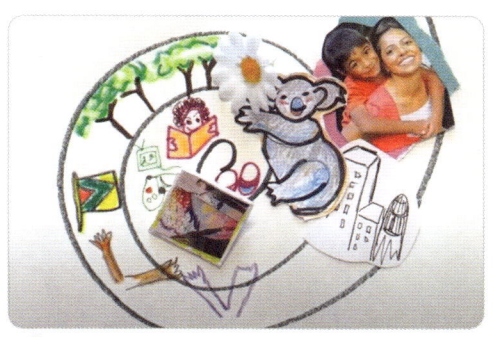

2. As you work outwards, add things that matter to you in the wider world. It could be wildlife, a place, or people who inspire you.

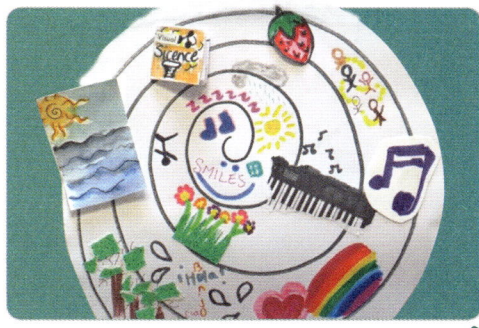

3. There's no right or wrong way to do this. It's your swirl, so what you choose to include and what it looks like is entirely up to you.

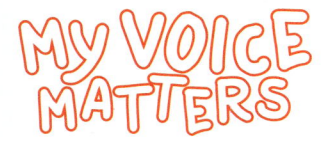

MY VOICE MATTERS

GET INSPIRED
Watch Place2Be's video for more tips
bit.ly/twi-swirl

Mental wellbeing

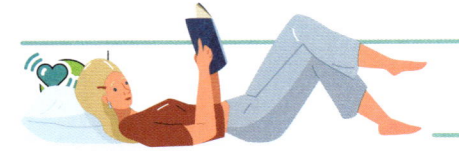

Find your happy place

Create a special space to feel happy and relaxed.

Your bedroom could be your happy place.

PLEASED PEOPLE
Finland is the happiest place in the world, according to the World Happiness Report 2023.

When you're feeling worried, sad or fed up it helps to have a place you can visit that helps you to feel better.

What is a happy place?
Your "happy place" can be a physical space – like your bedroom, a nearby park or your local library – or it can be a mental space, somewhere you think about that helps you feel calm. It could be somewhere you went on holiday, say, or a friend or a relative's home, or somewhere in your imagination. Your happy place could also refer to something you enjoy doing. For example, you might be in your happy place when you're reading, drawing or playing music. Your happy place is simply a place or situation where you feel comfortable, safe and happy, whether you are there physically or just in your imagination.

Music could be your happy place.

When to visit your happy place
Mindfulness teacher Frances Trussell says you can go to your happy place whenever you like. "A happy place is there for you whenever you might need it, especially if challenging feelings like fear, anger, anxiety or sadness arise and you want to feel calmer. Creating or identifying your happy place is a fantastic way to activate your imagination in a way that helps calm you." Your happy place is where you can take care of yourself – for example, by drawing or listening to your favourite songs. It's where you can go, even if it's in your mind, when you've had an argument or you are disappointed with exam results – or things just feel a bit much.

Create your own happy place
You can create your happy place and make it look and feel how you want. If you wanted to make your happy place in a corner of your bedroom you could make it comfy and cosy with cushions, a blanket, favourite toys, books or crafts. If your happy place is somewhere else, for example your grandparents' kitchen, you could take photos and make a collage. To invent a happy place in your mind, begin by thinking of a time when you felt happy, content and peaceful, or picture a place where you would feel like that. Describe that scene to yourself in detail so you can really imagine yourself there and you can recall it easily any time.

"I sit on the sand and chill"

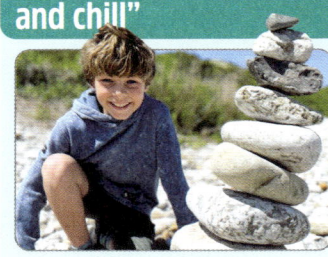

"My happy place is at the beach because when I go there I get to relax and maybe play cricket with my friends. Another reason I like going is to throw a Frisbee to my dog, Barney, who runs around like the Flash trying to catch it. I've recently learned how to skim stones and I spend a lot of my time practising. However, sometimes I prefer to just sit on the sand and chill."
Taylor, aged 12

Tips to visit a happy place in your mind

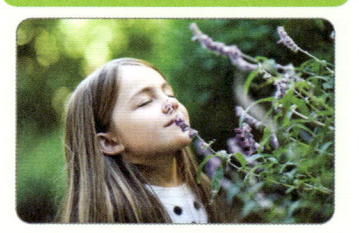

- Use a physical object, such as holding a pebble.
- Sniff a scent, such as lavender or chocolate, which reminds you of the place.
- Write a description of the happy place – the sight, sounds, smell and feel of it – to read and remind yourself.
- Record yourself reading the description so you can listen and imagine yourself there.

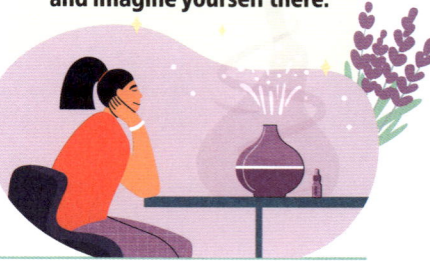

Find your happy place

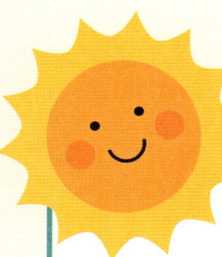

Draw a picture of your happy place.
What do you see?

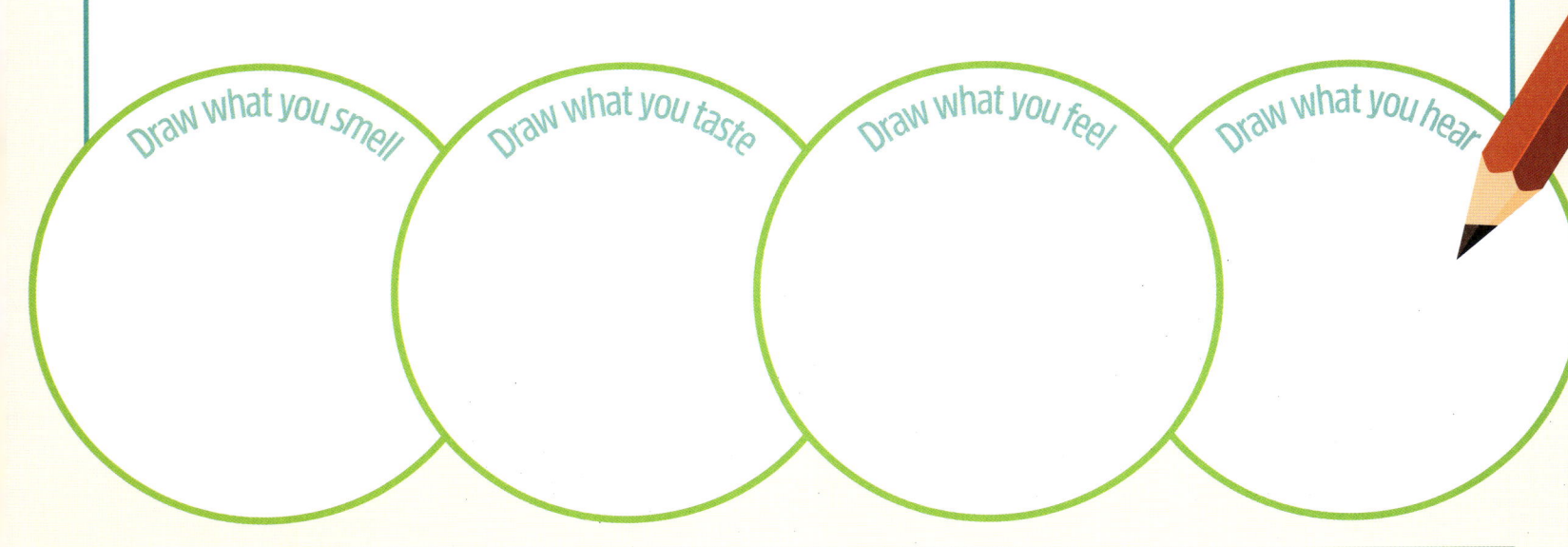

Draw what you smell

Draw what you taste

Draw what you feel

Draw what you hear

Mental wellbeing

It's good to talk

Conversation helps you understand and connect with others.

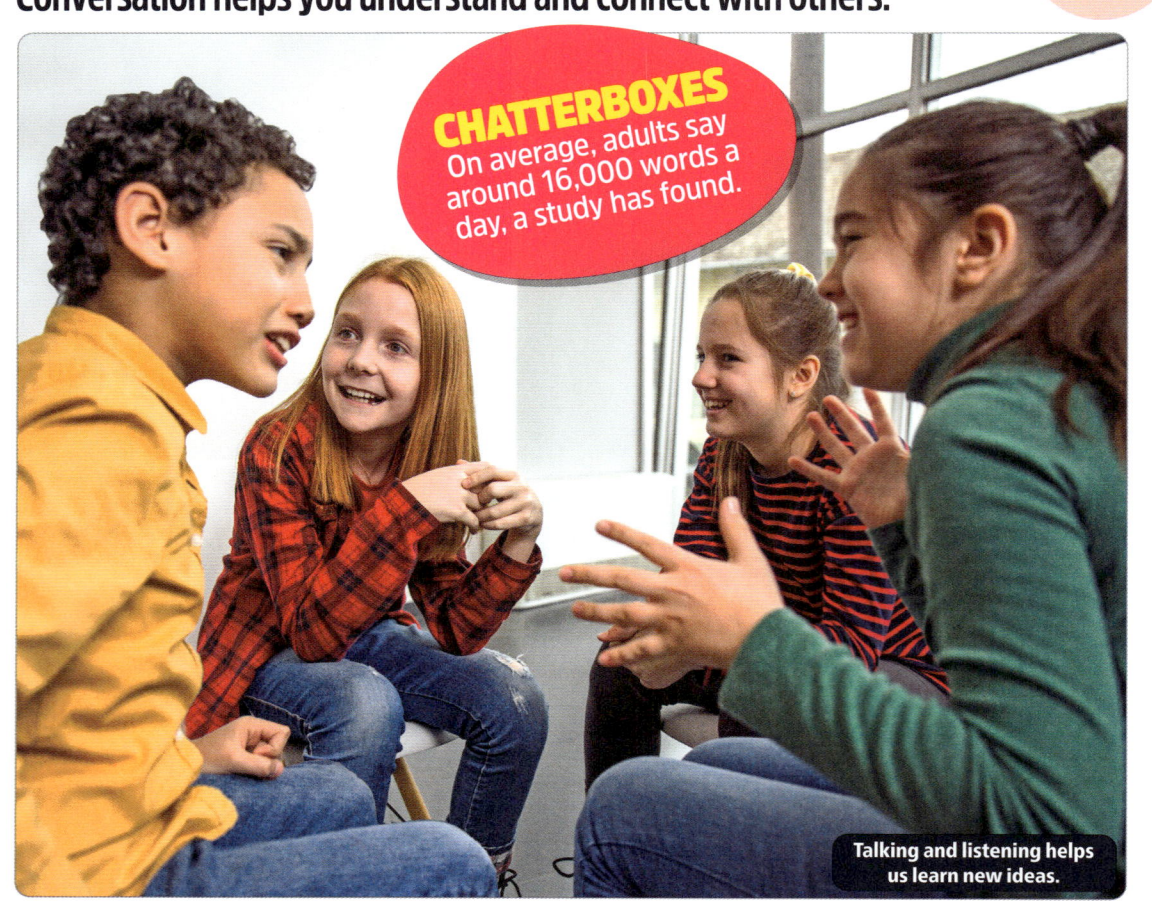

"I like texting and using emojis. They're fun."

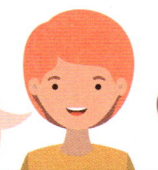

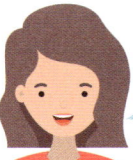

"Me too, but it's nice to talk as well."

CHATTERBOXES
On average, adults say around 16,000 words a day, a study has found.

Talking and listening helps us learn new ideas.

How to help conversations flow

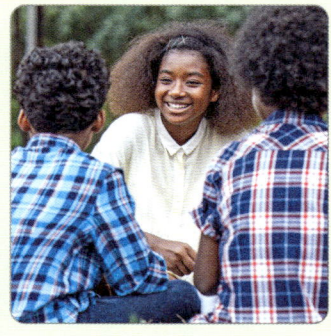

- Think about what you want to say and make it clear and easy to follow.
- Ask questions that need more than a "yes" or "no" answer. For example, start questions with the words why, how or what.
- Smile and nod while speaking and keep eye contact if you can.

Tips for listening well

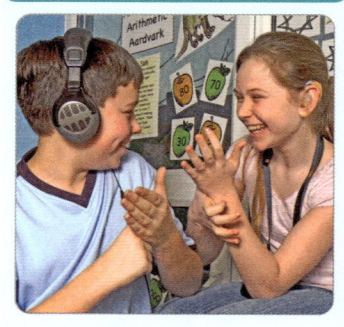

- When someone tells you something, repeat it back to show you're listening.
- Let them speak and try not to interrupt even if you want to share an idea or opinion.
- If your friend stops talking, wait a moment before speaking. They might be trying to find the right words to continue.

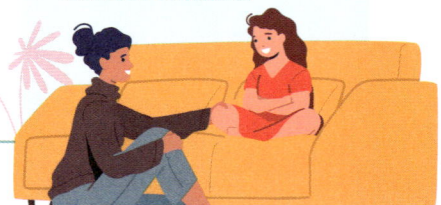

Have you ever been stuck for words? Knowing what to say and when to say it isn't always easy – but everyone can learn, practise and improve their communication skills.

What does communication mean?
Communication is how we share information and connect with others. We do it in lots of ways. When you have a conversation with someone you're not just swapping words. You are also expressing yourself through your tone of voice (how quietly or loudly you're speaking and the mood that suggests) and the way you move your face and body, known as body language. Conversation skills include starting conversations, using eye contact, knowing what to talk about and taking turns to speak and listen.

The benefits of conversation
Having a conversation where everyone gets the chance to speak and listen is great for sharing thoughts and feelings. Listening helps you to discover new ideas and develop empathy (understanding how other people are feeling) because you are seeing things through someone else's eyes.

Radio presenter Emma Barnett says that of all the many different ways we communicate – including text messages and emojis – talking gets across your message best because it's easier to understand what someone really means. Good communication opens up understanding, feeling and emotion, says Barnett.

Radio presenter Emma Barnett.

What makes good conversation?
A conversation involves taking turns to talk. Some people have a lot to say; others need encouragement to speak, so make sure everyone has a chance to join in. Listen carefully to what the other person is saying and don't be afraid to ask questions or share your opinion. Body language sends out messages about how we feel, so make sure you look at someone while speaking to them. If you see them nodding and smiling, this means they're showing interest. If they are yawning or turning away it could mean they've tuned out of the conversation. Advice expert Annalisa Barbieri believes listening is the most important part of conversation, and not just to someone's words but the way they say them. "It's about paying attention," she says.

It's good to talk

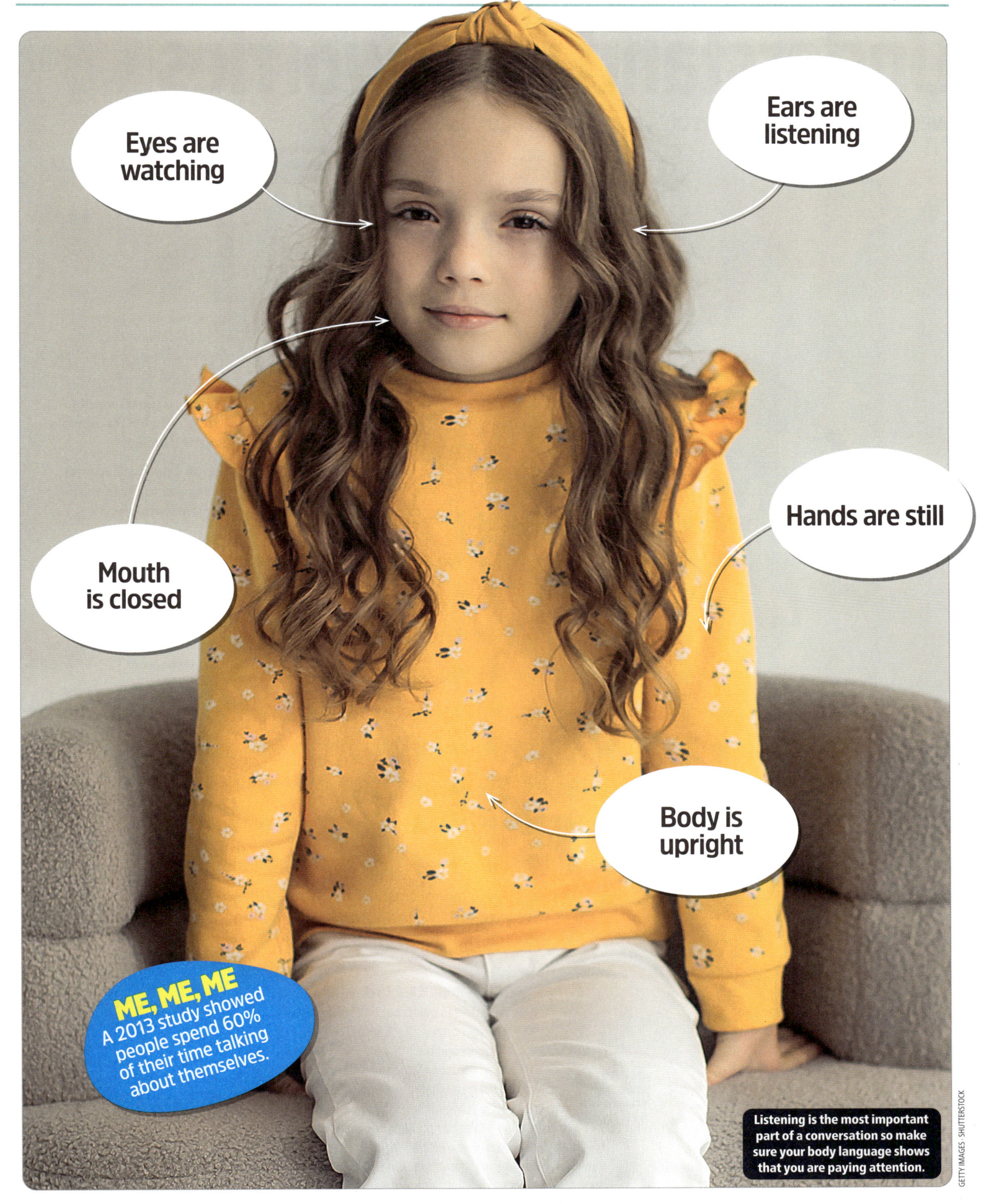

Eyes are watching

Ears are listening

Mouth is closed

Hands are still

Body is upright

ME, ME, ME
A 2013 study showed people spend 60% of their time talking about themselves.

Listening is the most important part of a conversation so make sure your body language shows that you are paying attention.

Mental wellbeing

Understand your worries

Everyone worries sometimes but you can turn it into positive action.

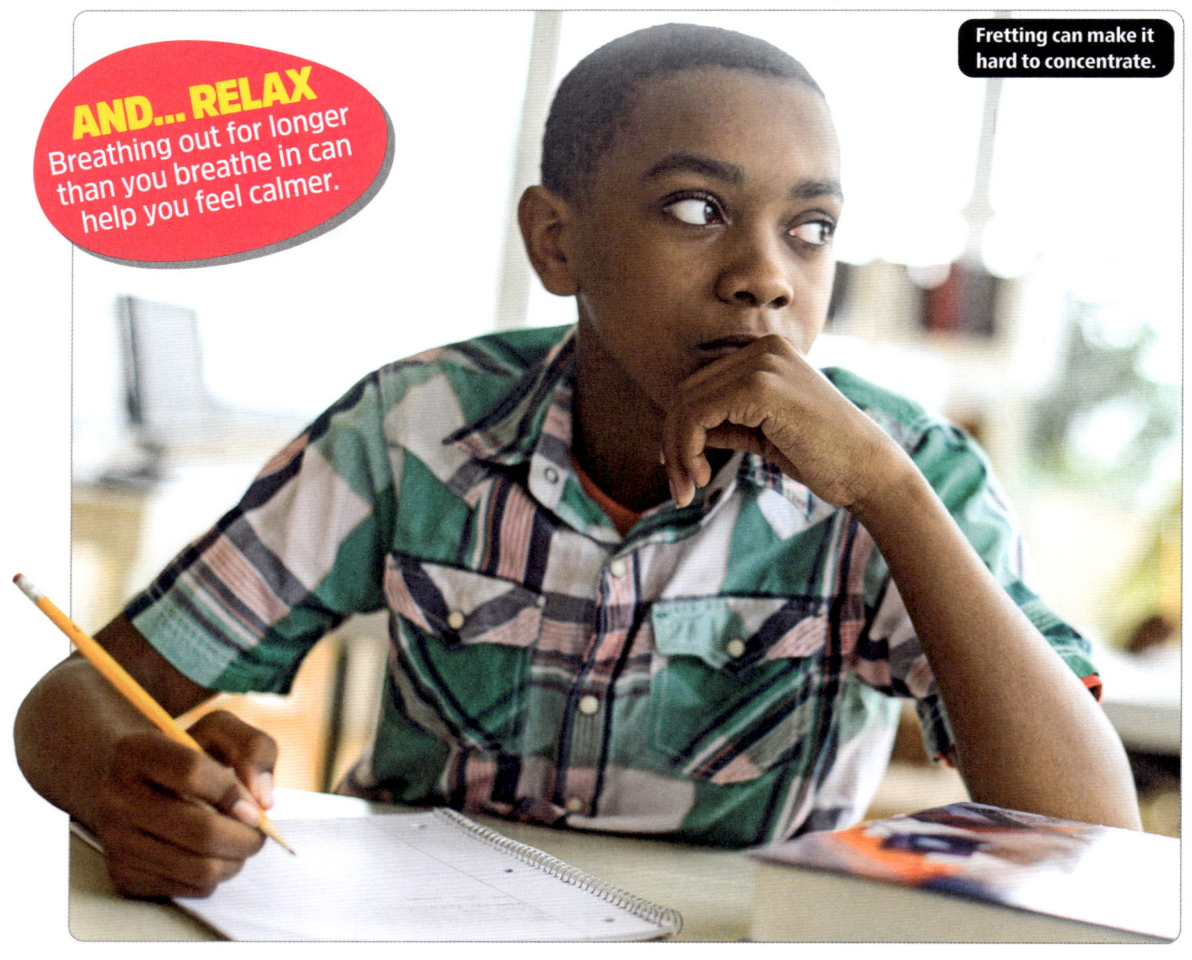

AND... RELAX Breathing out for longer than you breathe in can help you feel calmer.

Fretting can make it hard to concentrate.

Calm your worries

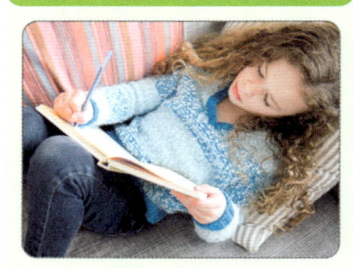

Young person's counsellor Angela McMillan suggests more ways to help when you're "what if-ing".

- Listen to your favourite song. Focus on the words and the tune.
- Write down your worries. Then you can keep the paper or tear it into shreds.
- Talk to a trusted adult or friend about how you feel.
- Name five things you can see, four things you can hear, three you can touch, two you can smell and one thing you can taste.

"I breathe or cartwheel"

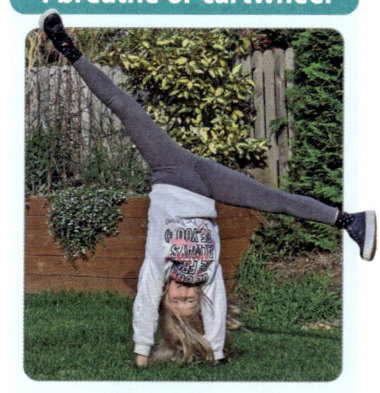

"When I have a "what-if" worry I sometimes do my seven-11 breathing. I breathe in while counting to seven and breathe out while counting to 11. This usually helps me to calm down and focus on something other than my worry. If this doesn't work, I like to do something physical, like dancing to Dua Lipa or cartwheeling."
Elodie, aged eight

It's common to wonder sometimes, "What if something goes wrong?" It's important to recognise that thought and manage it so that you don't get stuck in the worry.

What are "what if" thoughts?

Worrying about the future is a normal part of life. From time to time, everyone wonders what would happen if something doesn't go to plan: "What if I make a mistake?" or "What if everyone laughs at me?". These "what-if" worries focus on a negative outcome. When you spend a lot of time worrying about bad things that could happen, it's called "catastrophising" – because you're imagining the future could be a catastrophe. Spending a lot of time "what if-ing" makes you feel anxious and stressed. For example, you might feel tense and unwell, it might make you not want to do things, and it can make it hard to concentrate on what you're doing or what people are saying.

How to deal with the worries

There are different ways you can help yourself. Young person's counsellor Angela McMillan suggests creating an "If/then" plan. "For example," she says, "IF you have to stand up in front of the class, THEN you will take three deep breaths and remind yourself you have prepared and you're ok. Or IF the social event is really noisy and you feel overwhelmed, THEN you can step outside for a few minutes." You can also identify what you're worrying about and then challenge it. Ask yourself how likely it is to actually happen. Try thinking about what could go right. For example, instead of thinking "What if I miss the ball when I try to kick it?" flip that around to ask "What if I kick the ball on target?"

Be kind to yourself.

It's important to be kind

McMillan points out that most worries never happen. "Remember they are thoughts and the bravest thing we can do is to not let the worry win," she says. Try to focus your attention on what you're doing. That could be the book you're reading, the TV show you're watching or the conversation you're having. Getting cross with yourself will make you feel worse, so be kind to yourself. Think about how you would talk to a friend who is feeling worried – and then speak to yourself in that same way.

90

Understand your worries

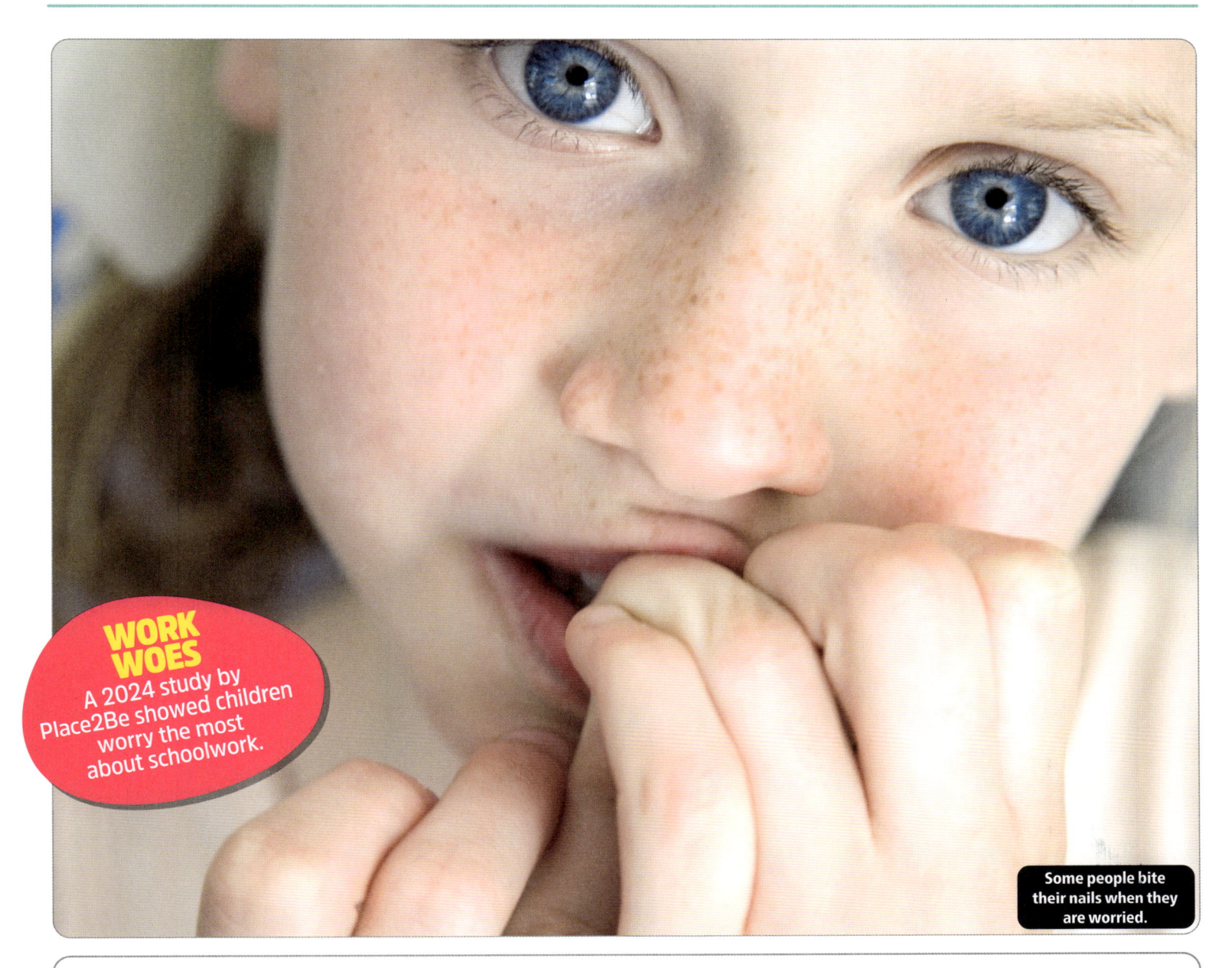

WORK WOES
A 2024 study by Place2Be showed children worry the most about schoolwork.

Some people bite their nails when they are worried.

IF... Fill in your If/then plan: **THEN...**

Mental wellbeing

The fidget factor

Twiddling your thumbs and tapping your feet can make you less stressed.

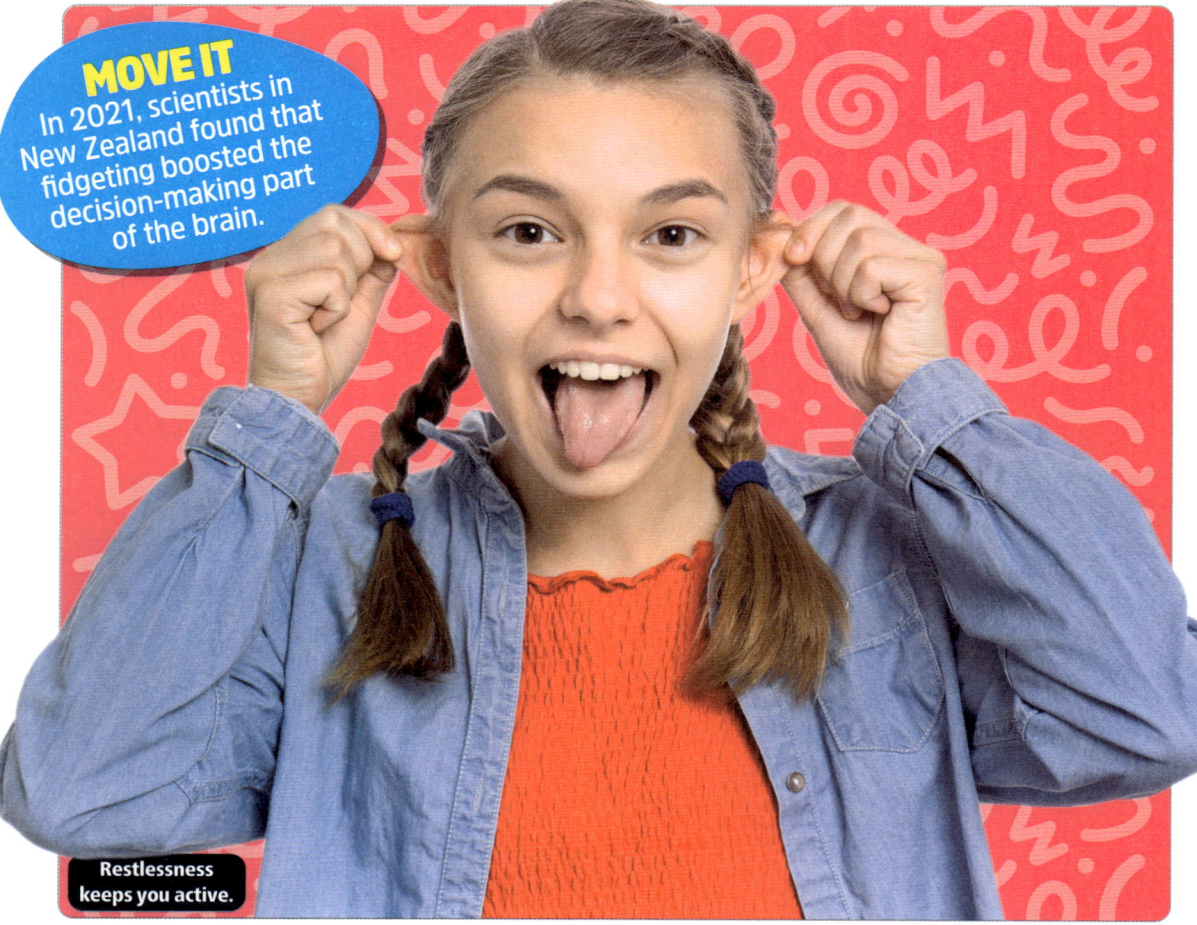

MOVE IT
In 2021, scientists in New Zealand found that fidgeting boosted the decision-making part of the brain.

Restlessness keeps you active.

Fidgeting is often seen as a sign of being bored or restless. Some might think you're not paying attention but studies show that having ants in your pants could be good for you.

What is fidgeting?
Fidgeting means making small, restless movements without meaning to. It can be soothing and repetitive, like drumming your fingers on a desk, or feeling the need to shuffle around in your chair because you can't get comfy. Do you often find yourself tapping your toes, jiggling your knees, nibbling your nails or twiddling your hair? Most people, including grown-ups, get the fidgets from time to time and scientists say people are more likely to fidget when they are excited, worried or tired, but it can happen any time.

How is it good for you?
Have you ever felt restless on a long car journey or while watching a film? Scientists say this could be our body's way of telling us to move around and burn energy. As well as keeping you fit, fidgeting has been shown to reduce stress. It also gets your brain going, explains scientist Anne Churchland. Some people need to be calm and still to think, but for others twisting and twiddling boosts their concentration and memory. "Fidgeting actually helps many of us to relax, focus and tackle tasks," Churchland says.

Knitting can be very relaxing.

Find your fidget
Moving around when you need to sit still – for instance, in class – can disturb others as well as yourself, so it's good to fidget responsibly. Research shows that doodling (drawing pictures or patterns while thinking of something else) can improve concentration and help you remember more information. Playing with putty or squeezing a stress ball can help you stay calm and focused. Author Dr Kat Arney says some forms of deliberate fidgeting, like knitting, can be very relaxing. Everyone unwinds in different ways, so whether it's playing a musical instrument or making crafts while watching TV, try to find the best fidget for you.

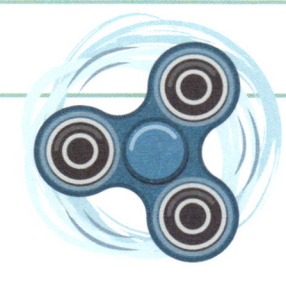

Ideas from a reader

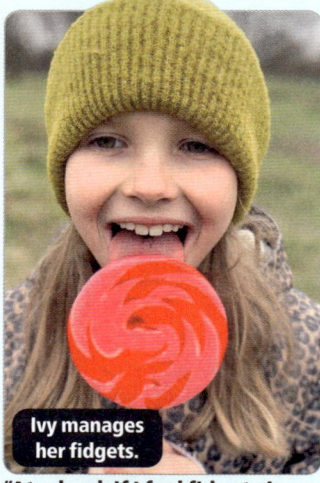

Ivy manages her fidgets.

"At school, if I feel fidgety in class I try to concentrate really hard and put my hands flat on the desk to help me focus. At home, when I watch TV, I like to do more than one thing or I get fidgety. So I'll get some LEGO or do origami paper things to help me stay still." Ivy, aged nine

Why not make your own fidget ball?

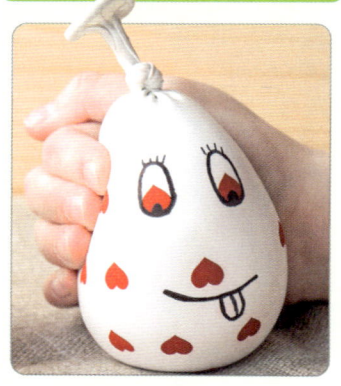

Carefully fill a balloon with flour, dried rice or small beads until it's about the size of your fist. Squeeze out all the air and tightly tie the top. Decorate your fidget ball by tying some wool around the top to make hair and draw happy, angry or funny faces with a marker pen. Then next time you're feeling restless, squeeze!

The fidget factor

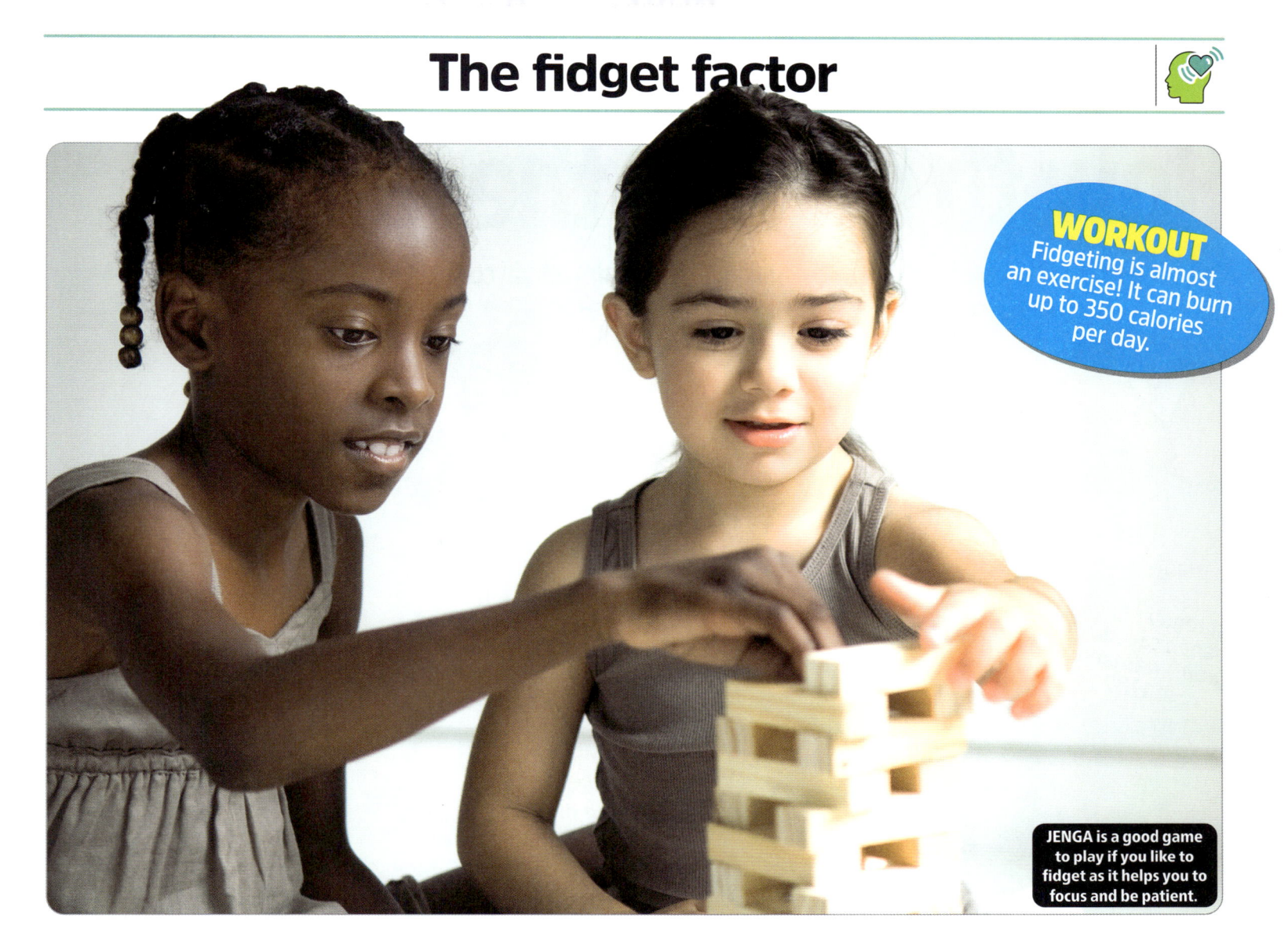

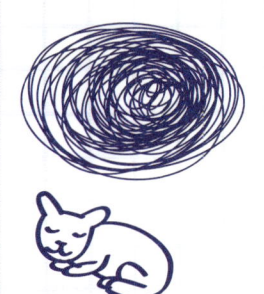

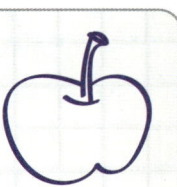

WORKOUT
Fidgeting is almost an exercise! It can burn up to 350 calories per day.

JENGA is a good game to play if you like to fidget as it helps you to focus and be patient.

Doodle here when you're bored:

93

Mental wellbeing

How to handle the news

Learning to cope with lots of news can make you feel calm and in control.

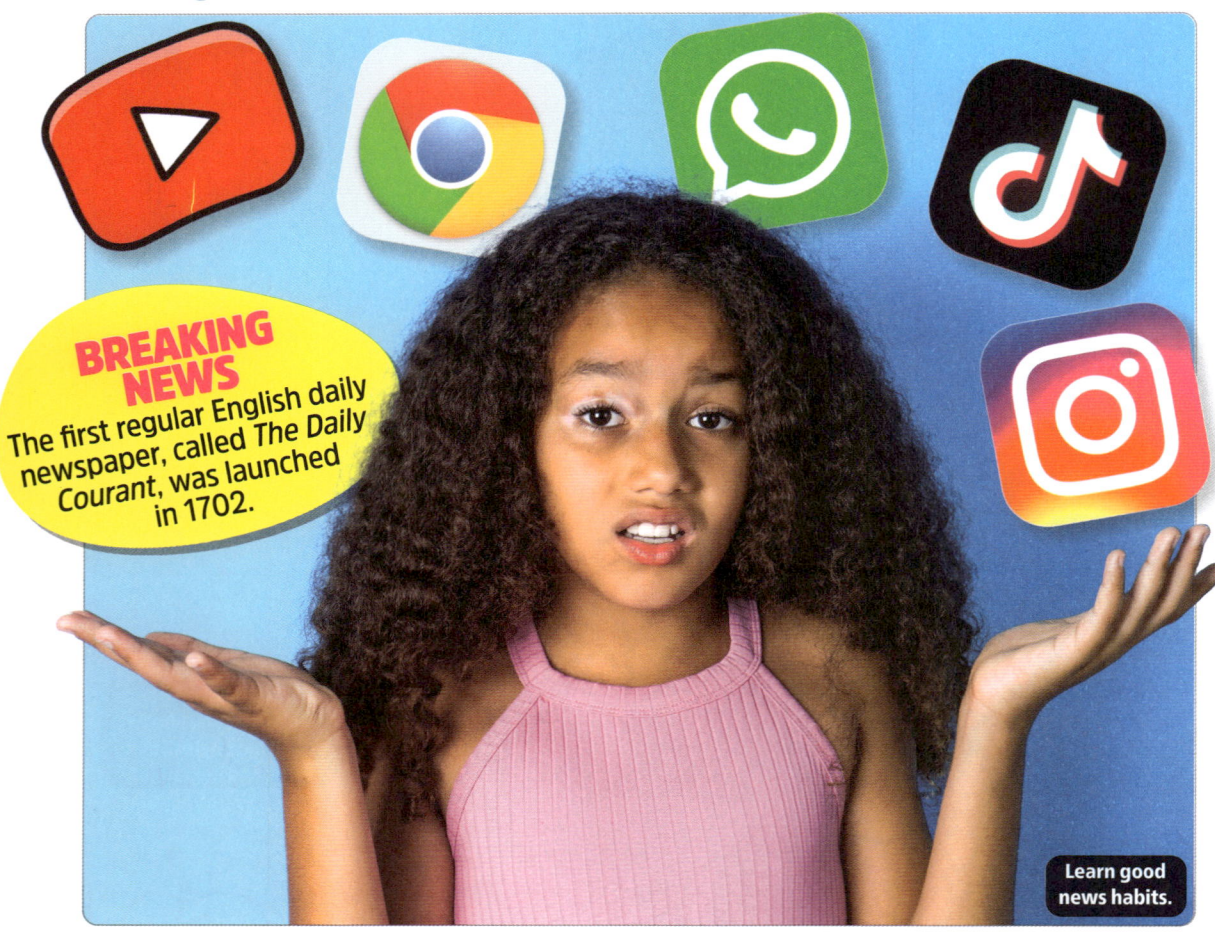

BREAKING NEWS
The first regular English daily newspaper, called *The Daily Courant*, was launched in 1702.

Learn good news habits.

Top tips to deal with too much news

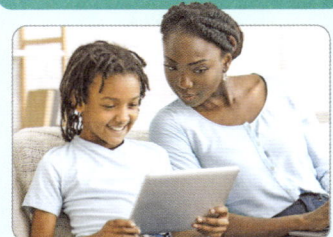

- Only read a few stories at a time and talk about them to someone afterwards.
- Focus on life away from the news and stick to familiar routines, like going to sports practice or meeting friends.
- If a friend is upset by the news, talk it over with them.

Find more top tips and advice at theweekjunior.co.uk/advice

Take action to help with climate worries

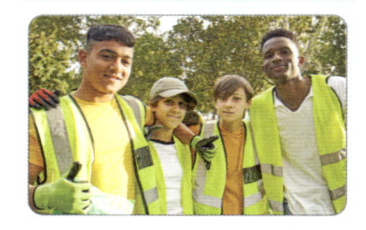

- **Make it fun**
Set up a climate club with friends and organise activities like litter-picking, making posters that encourage recycling and setting up a book swap.
- **Focus on good news**
Lots of people are working on solutions to climate change. Set a challenge to find one positive climate story each week.
- **Take action**
Everyone can do something to make our world a better place. Learn how to be an energy hero here: tinyurl.com/TWJ-Energyhero

News is all around us and it's normal to feel a little bit anxious when you see stories that seem worrying. There are positive steps you can take to help with your feelings.

Where does news come from?
News reports come from many sources all over the world. As well as newspapers and magazines like *The Week Junior*, news is reported on television, radio and websites, and shared on social media. Stories grab the headlines for several reasons, including how unexpected they are and the number of people they affect. Stories like, say, what is happening in Israel, or a big earthquake, often appear as rolling news. This means the reports are updated frequently, talked about and shared. Being surrounded by news like this can make you feel the events are part of your life, no matter how far away they actually are.

How does news affect you?
It's interesting and fun to learn about inspiring and uplifting stories, but bad news happens too, and reports about war or climate change can make you feel angry, anxious or upset. "Bad news isn't nice to hear," says psychotherapist Dr Aaron Balick (an expert on thoughts and feelings). "People are suffering and there are real risks. It is normal to feel worried about these things." Studies also show that we're more likely to notice bad news stories and remember them more clearly than positive ones. This is called "negativity bias" and scientists say it's a very old survival technique that keeps us safe and alert to danger.

Look out for positive stories.

How can you cope with worrying news?
It's important to listen to facts rather than rumours, Balick explains. If you're alarmed by a story you've heard about on social media, for example, ask an adult to help you check it on a reliable news website like BBC News. Another way to deal with difficult news is to put your worry into action. If you find stories about climate change upsetting, write to your MP and tell them your concerns. Also, don't keep your feelings to yourself, says Balick. Talk to a trusted adult, because this may help you understand where your emotions come from and why you feel this way.

How to handle the news

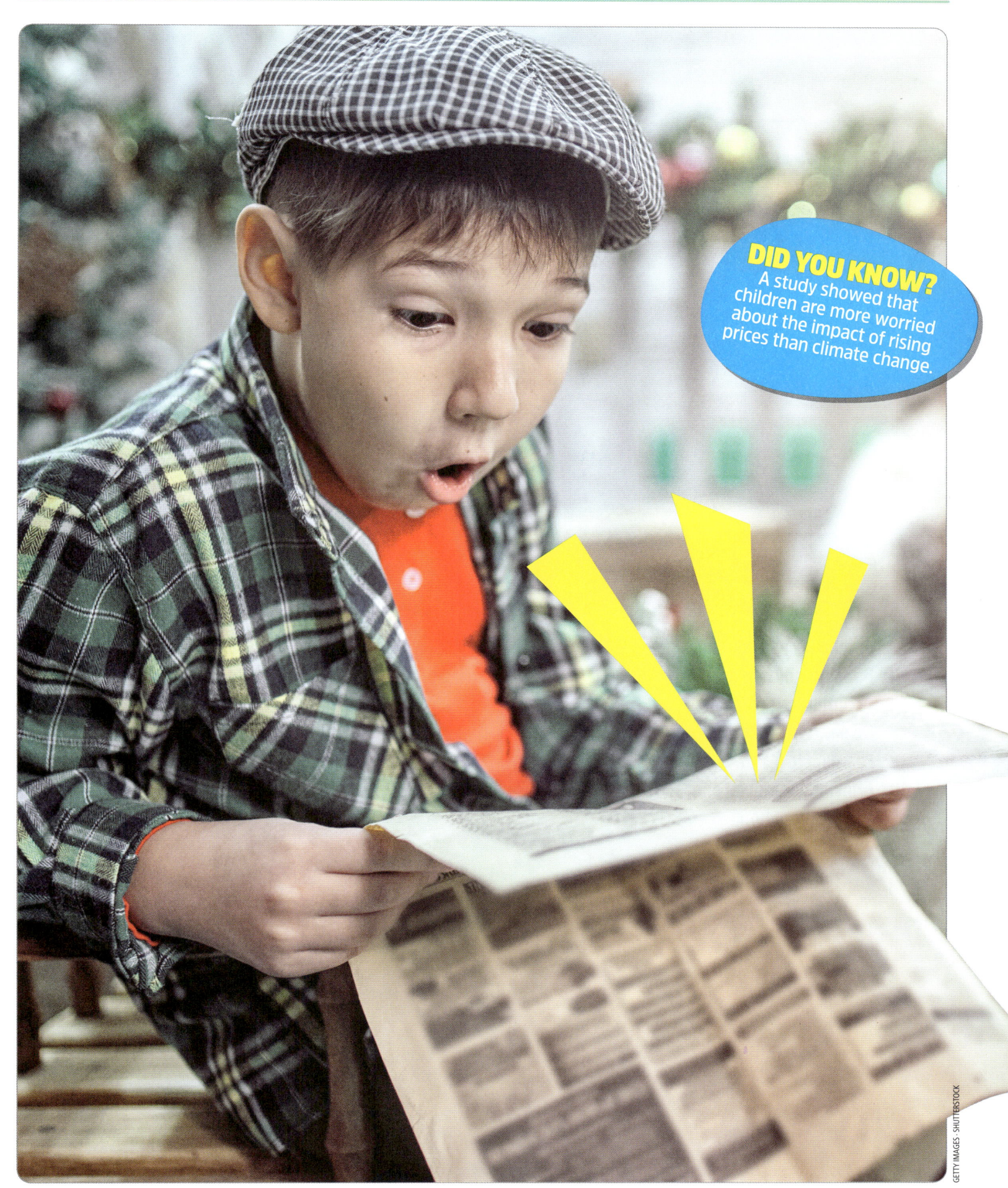

DID YOU KNOW? A study showed that children are more worried about the impact of rising prices than climate change.

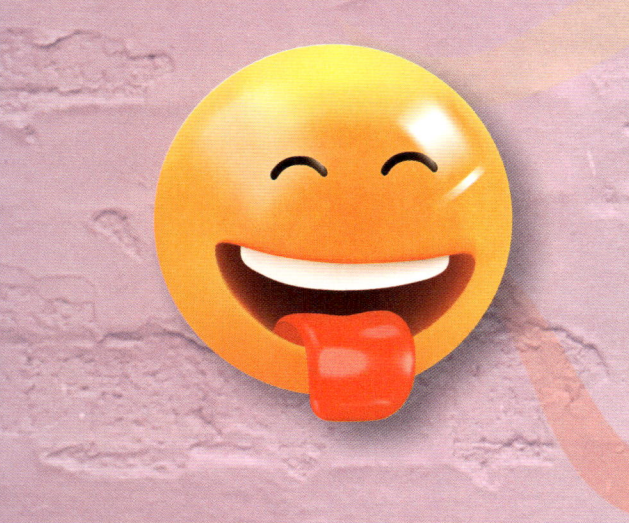

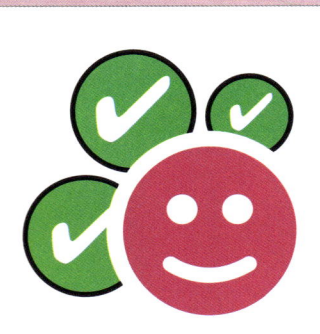

- **98** Spread joy with kindness
- **100** Put empathy into action
- **102** Accepting tricky feelings
- **104** Dealing with drama
- **106** Learning to let go
- **108** Grieving for a loved one
- **110** The power of hope

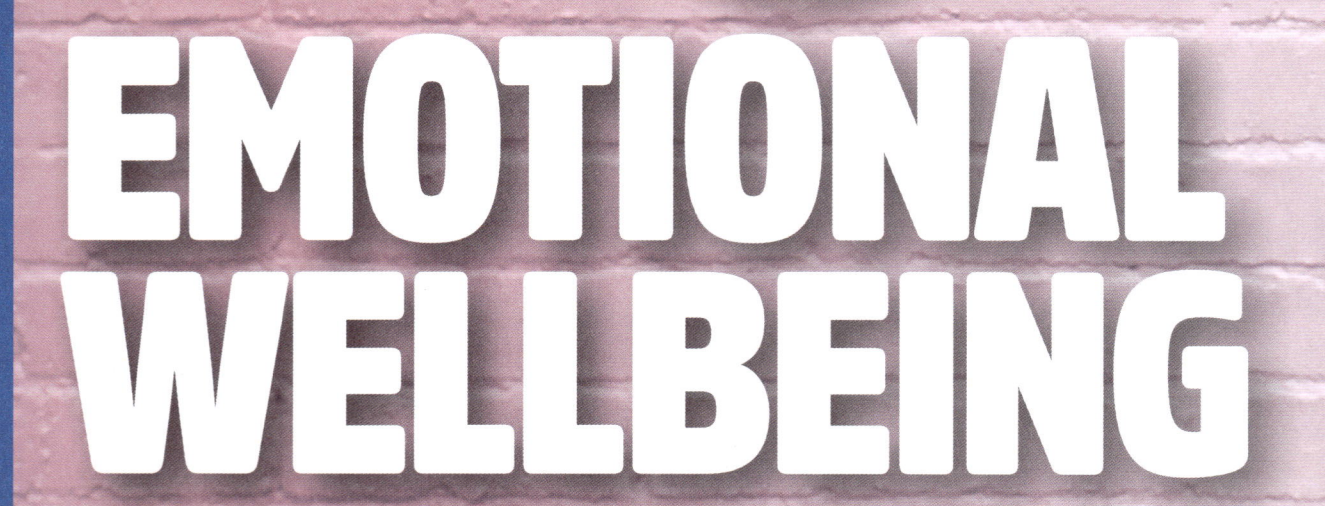

EMOTIONAL WELLBEING

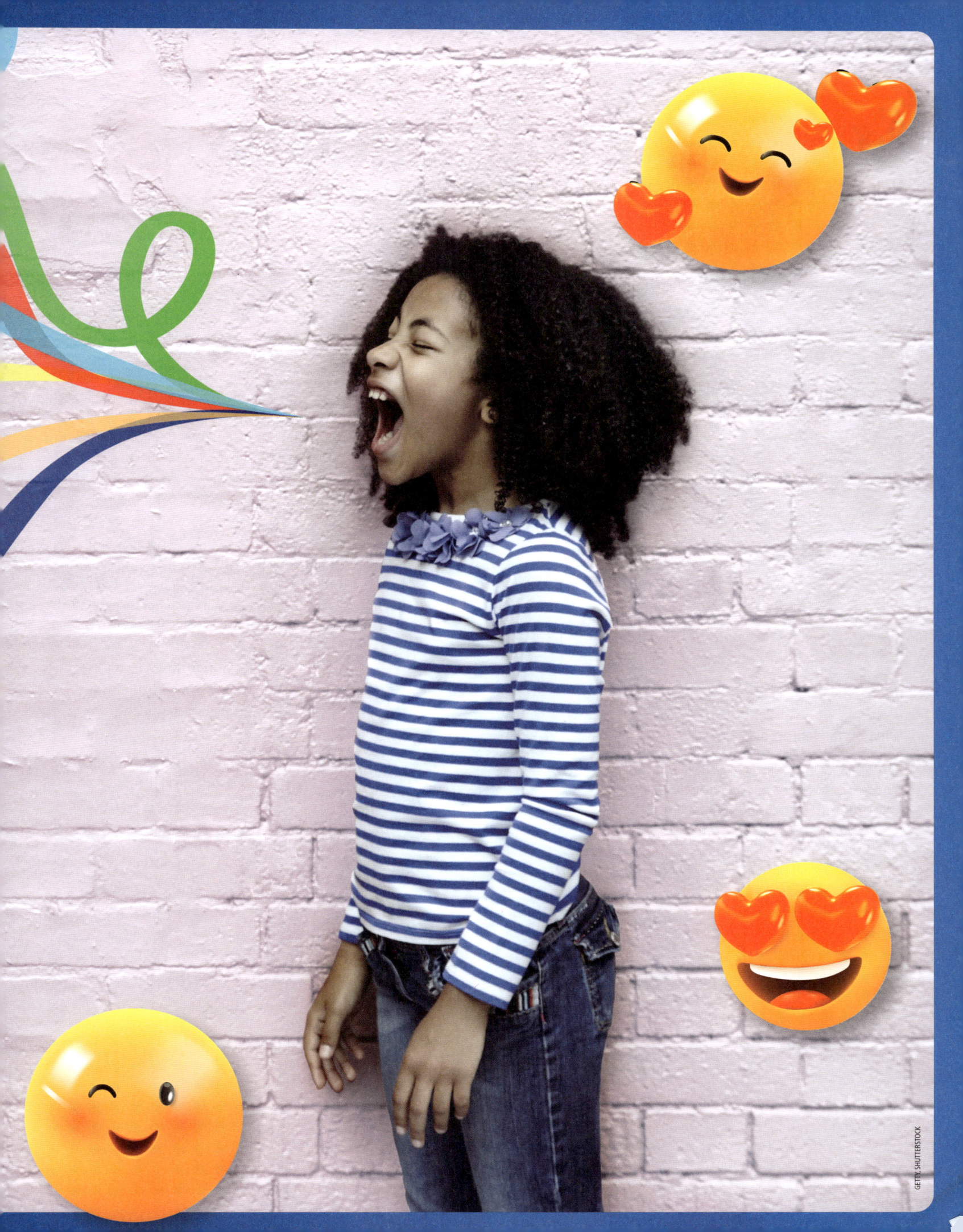

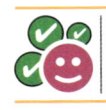

Emotional wellbeing

Spread joy with kindness
Helping others is not just a virtue but a positive force for good.

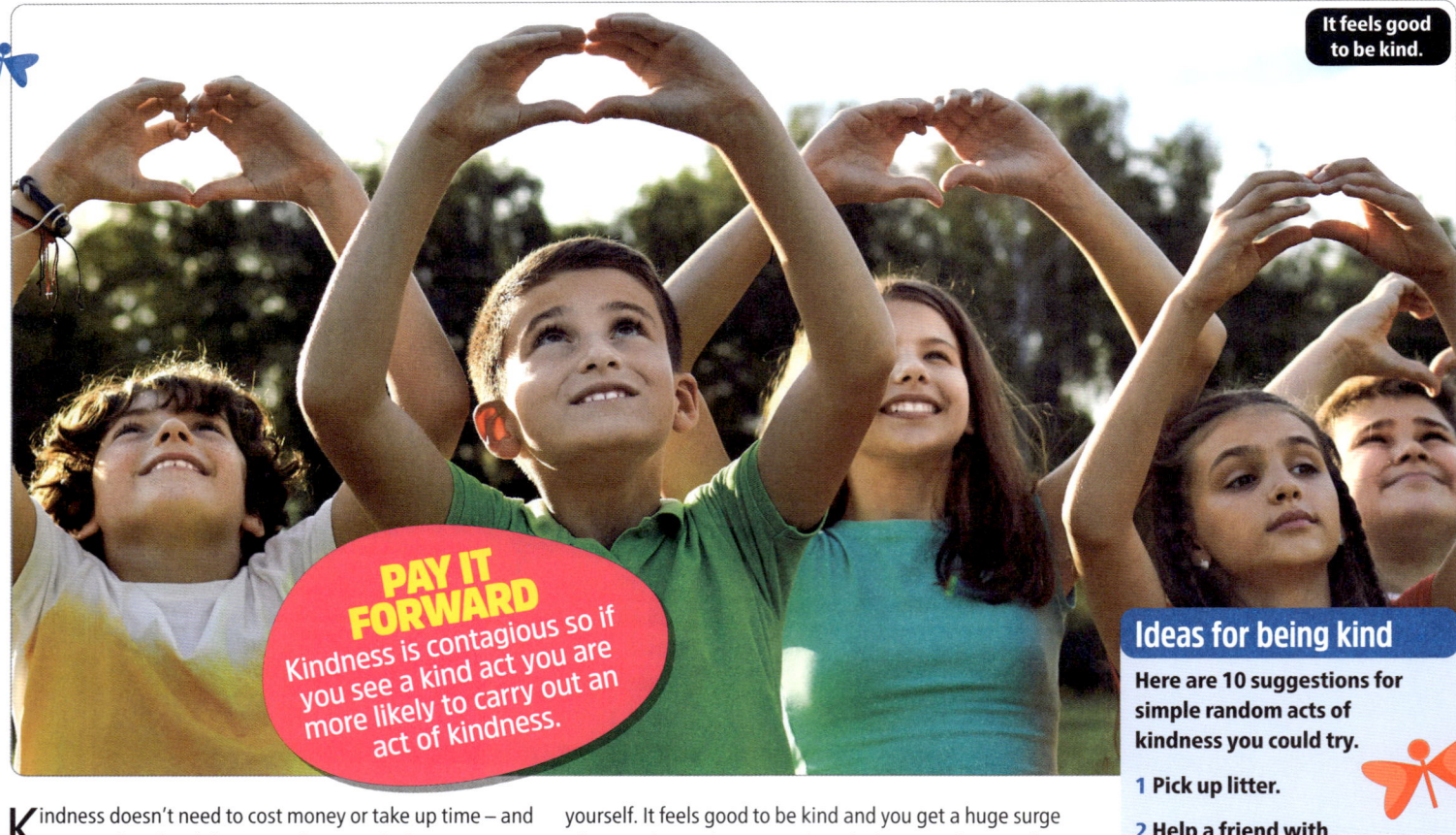

It feels good to be kind.

PAY IT FORWARD
Kindness is contagious so if you see a kind act you are more likely to carry out an act of kindness.

Kindness doesn't need to cost money or take up time – and it can make a big difference to how you feel.

What is a random act of kindness?
A random act of kindness is doing something for someone else without expecting to be rewarded for it. It refers to an unplanned positive action, and you do it for a friend or for a stranger.

Kindness is good for you
Everyone benefits from kindness – not only the person on the receiving end but also the person who carries out the kind act, as well as anyone watching it happen. Kindness is considered contagious (it spreads between people) because when you witness an act of kindness, you're more likely to go on to do something kind for another person yourself. Studies show that being kind can make you feel stronger, more energetic, more optimistic and happier. It can even reduce pain because of the chemicals it releases inside the body. Kindness is powerful.

Psychologist Suzy Reading highlights more benefits of practising kindness, "Being kind to other people is a great way to feel connected and it will help you feel positive about yourself. It feels good to be kind and you get a huge surge of energy from it but remember, the key is to do a good turn. You're not just doing it to make yourself feel good."

Different ways of being kind
You can demonstrate kindness anywhere – at home, at school, in your community, with your family or friends. The act can be unplanned, for example, if you notice someone drop their glove on the ground you could pick it up and give it back to them. You can look out for opportunities, too, such as holding a door open, paying someone a compliment or helping a teacher tidy up your classroom. You can also plan acts of kindness by drawing a picture for a friend, writing a note praising someone or donating old toys that you no longer play with to charity.

Suzy Reading suggests thinking about the people around you, "Who could do with a helping hand? Is there a friend that needs cheering up or could you include your brother or sister in your game? You can sprinkle some kindness around with a smile or a heartfelt thank you." Remember, what makes it a true act of kindness is doing it with no expectation of being thanked or getting anything in return.

Think about who needs cheering up.

Ideas for being kind
Here are 10 suggestions for simple random acts of kindness you could try.

1 Pick up litter.
2 Help a friend with their schoolwork.
3 Clean up after a meal.
4 Sort old clothes or toys and give them to charity.
5 Write a letter to a relative.
6 Offer to tidy up after class.
7 Give a friend a hug.
8 Lend a book to someone you think will enjoy it.
9 Tell someone that you appreciate them.
10 Make someone laugh.

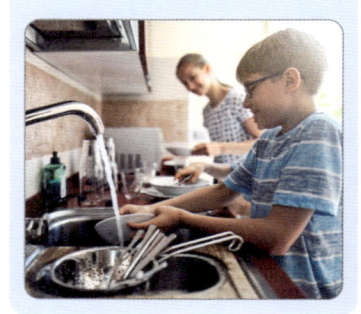

Spread joy with kindness

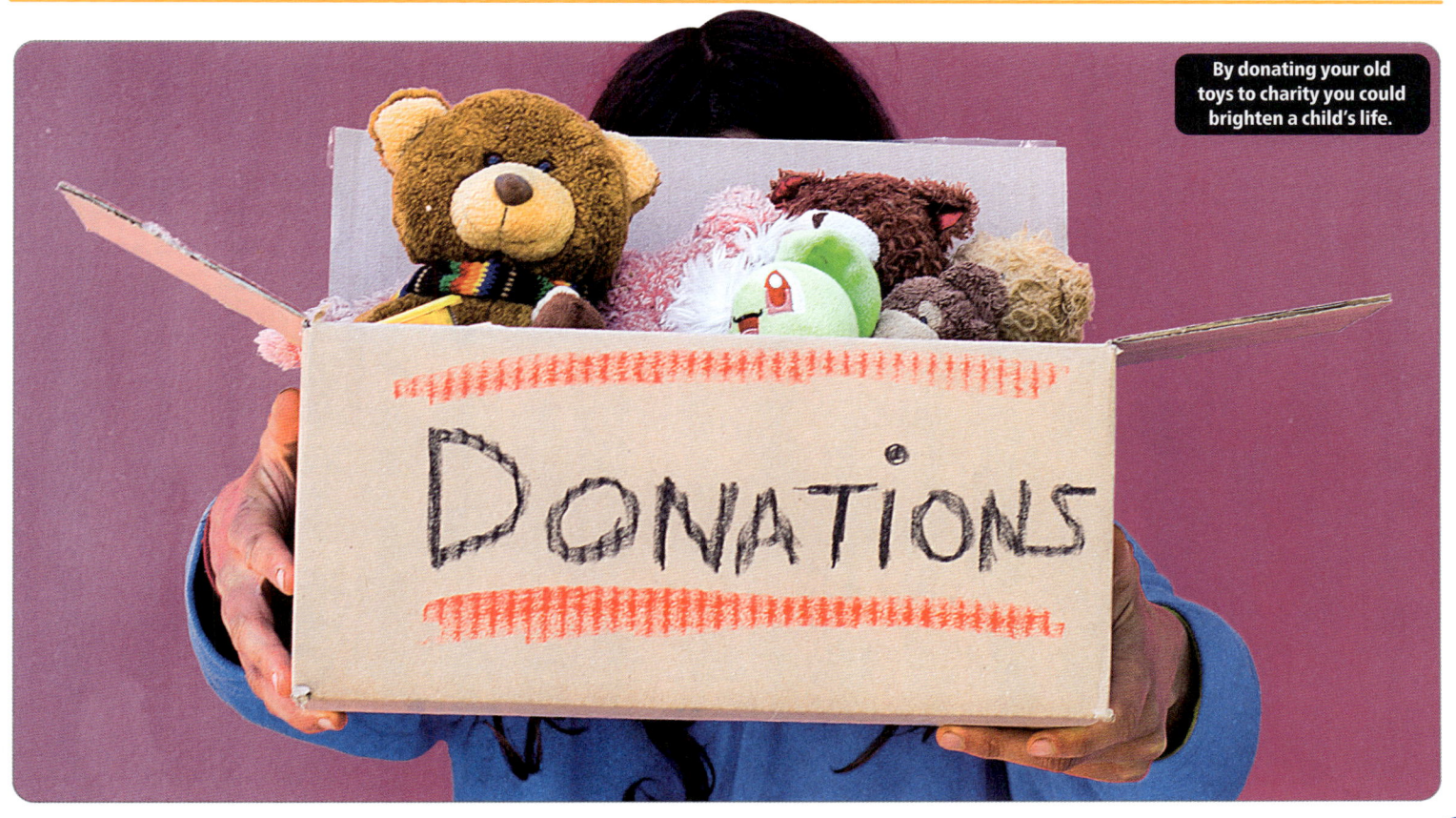

By donating your old toys to charity you could brighten a child's life.

I can show kindness by...

Write down random acts of kindness you could perform in the following columns:

HELPING:	SAYING:	DOING:

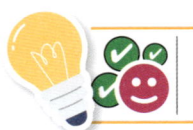

Emotional wellbeing
Put empathy into action
Understanding other people's feelings can build better friendships.

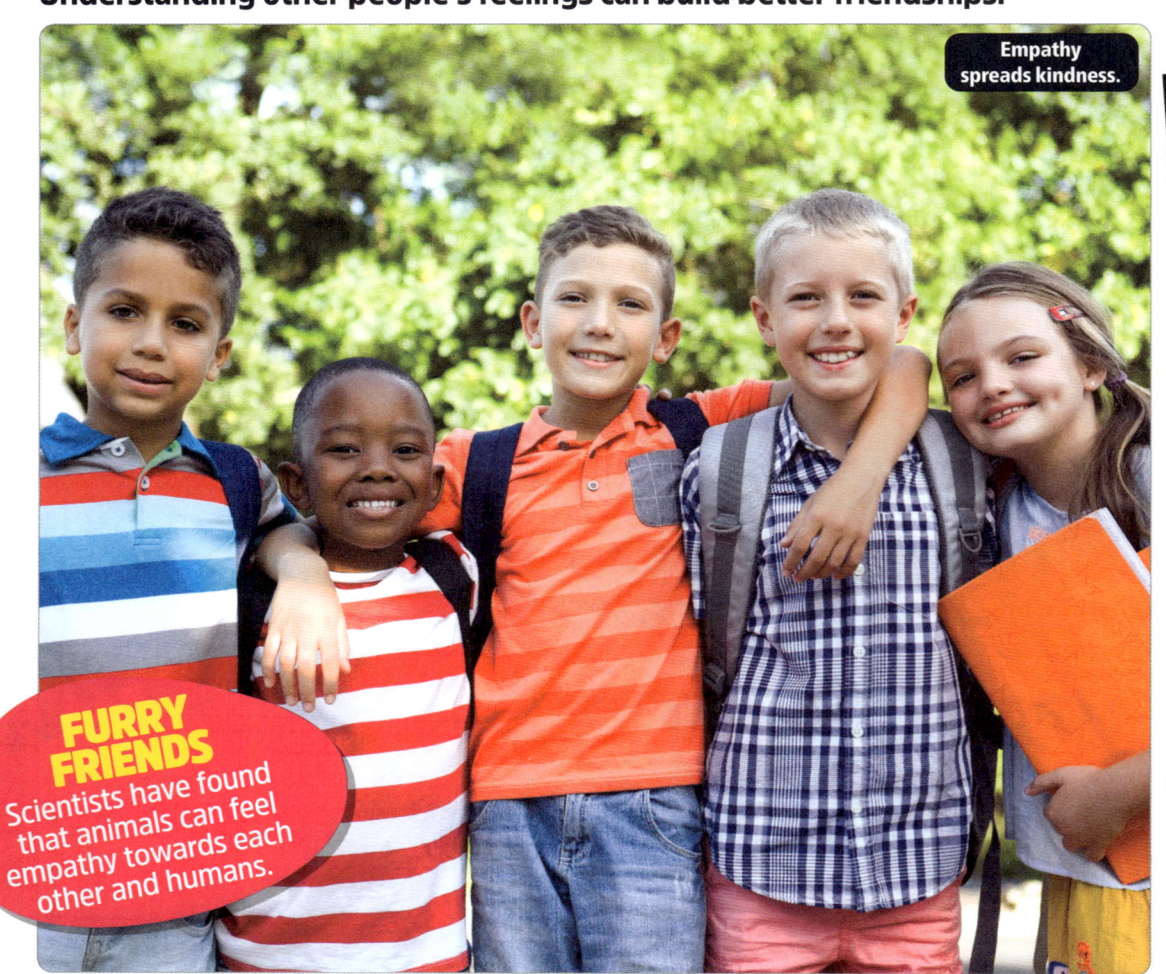

Empathy spreads kindness.

Five books to boost your empathy powers
- **Our Tower** by Joseph Coelho & Richard Johnson
- **Keep Dancing, Lizzie Chu** by Maisie Chan
- **Can You Feel the Noise?** By Stewart Foster
- **Let's Chase Stars Together: Poems to Lose Yourself In** by Matt Goodfellow
- **The Light in Everything** by Katya Balen

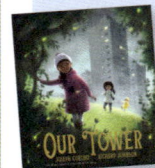

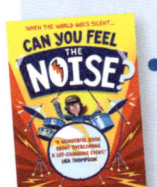

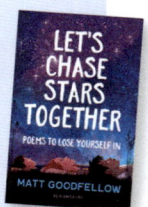

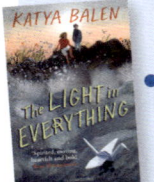

FURRY FRIENDS
Scientists have found that animals can feel empathy towards each other and humans.

Have you ever struggled to understand how someone else feels? Building up your empathy skills not only helps you connect with your friends, it also spreads kindness and inspires others to do the same.

What is empathy?
Empathy is a superpower that lets you step into someone else's shoes and understand how they feel. If you see your friend is upset after losing a football match, for example, and you support them, you are showing empathy. As well as making you a better friend, empathy inspires others to show kindness too. Miranda McKearney is from EmpathyLab, an organisation that builds empathy through reading. She believes even small actions can have a positive impact. "Empathy is a force for change," she says.

How can you have more empathy?
Scientists say empathy isn't something you are born with, it's a skill you learn. One way you can do this is by active listening. This is when you give someone your full attention when they're talking to you, listening closely and responding in a way that shows you understand. Reading is also a great way to boost empathy, because stories can take you inside someone else's mind and show you the world through their eyes and emotions.

Empathy helps you connect with others.

Putting empathy into action
Helen Riess, a psychiatrist (an expert on thoughts and feelings), recommends not just stepping into someone else's shoes but taking a walk in them. This could mean trying out something that is important to a friend or family member, like exploring their favourite place. EmpathyLab's Mission Empathy Challenge has ideas for putting empathy into action in schools or at home. That might be connecting with someone new in your class and having a friendly conversation, or making small changes to your behaviour. To find out more, visit empathylab.uk with an adult.

Tips for making an empathy resolution
- Think about what would make your home or school a happier, more caring place.
- Decide what you will do to make a difference.
- Make and share your resolution with your friends and family.
- Start acting on your resolution now.

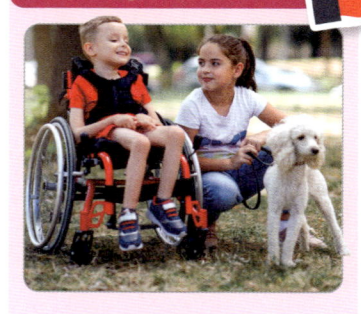

Put empathy into action

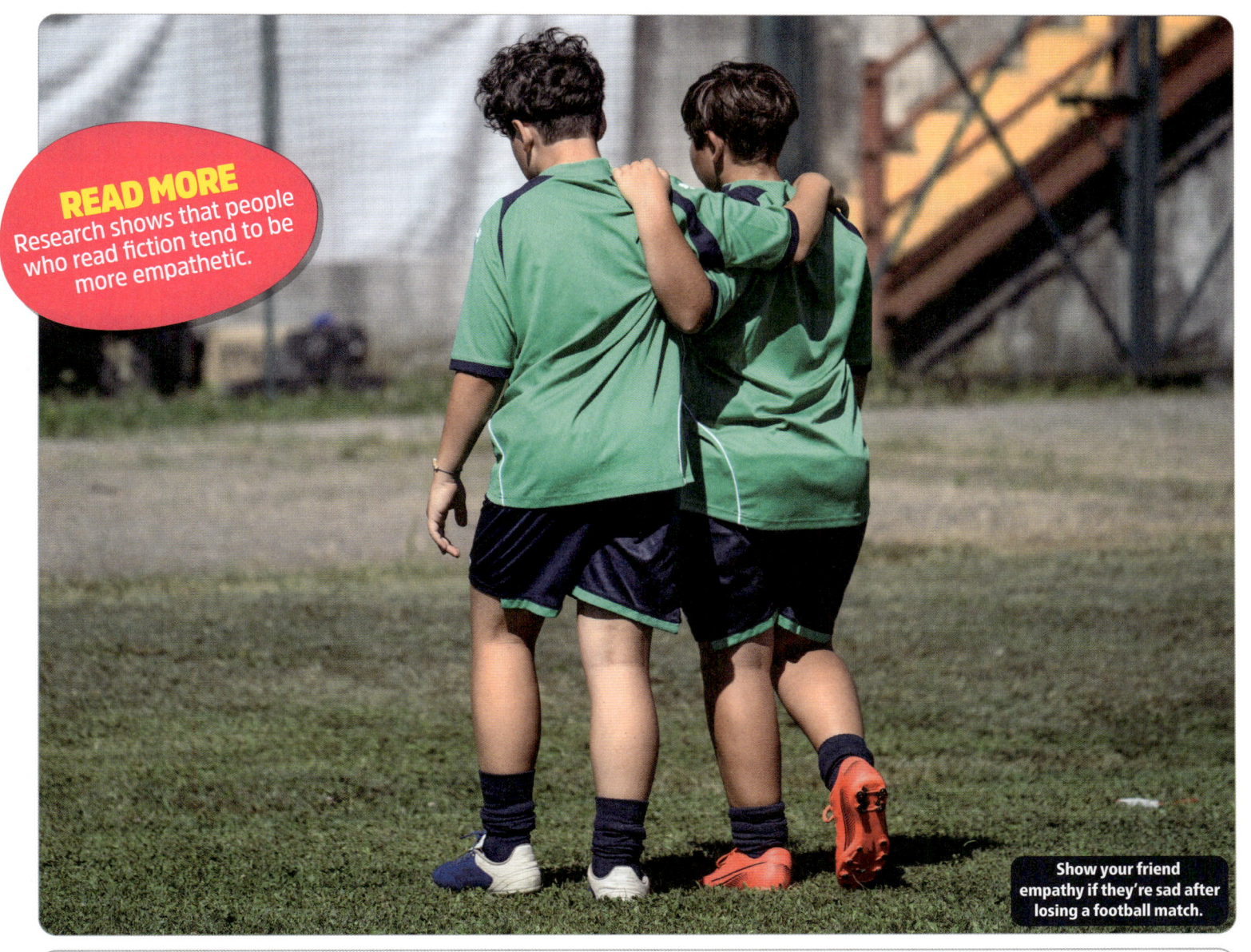

READ MORE
Research shows that people who read fiction tend to be more empathetic.

Show your friend empathy if they're sad after losing a football match.

Think about a situation where your friend may need empathy

What do you think your friend is feeling and why?

If you were in their situation what would you want your friends to say to you?

Emotional wellbeing

Accepting tricky feelings
Learning to understand uncomfortable emotions can bring you peace.

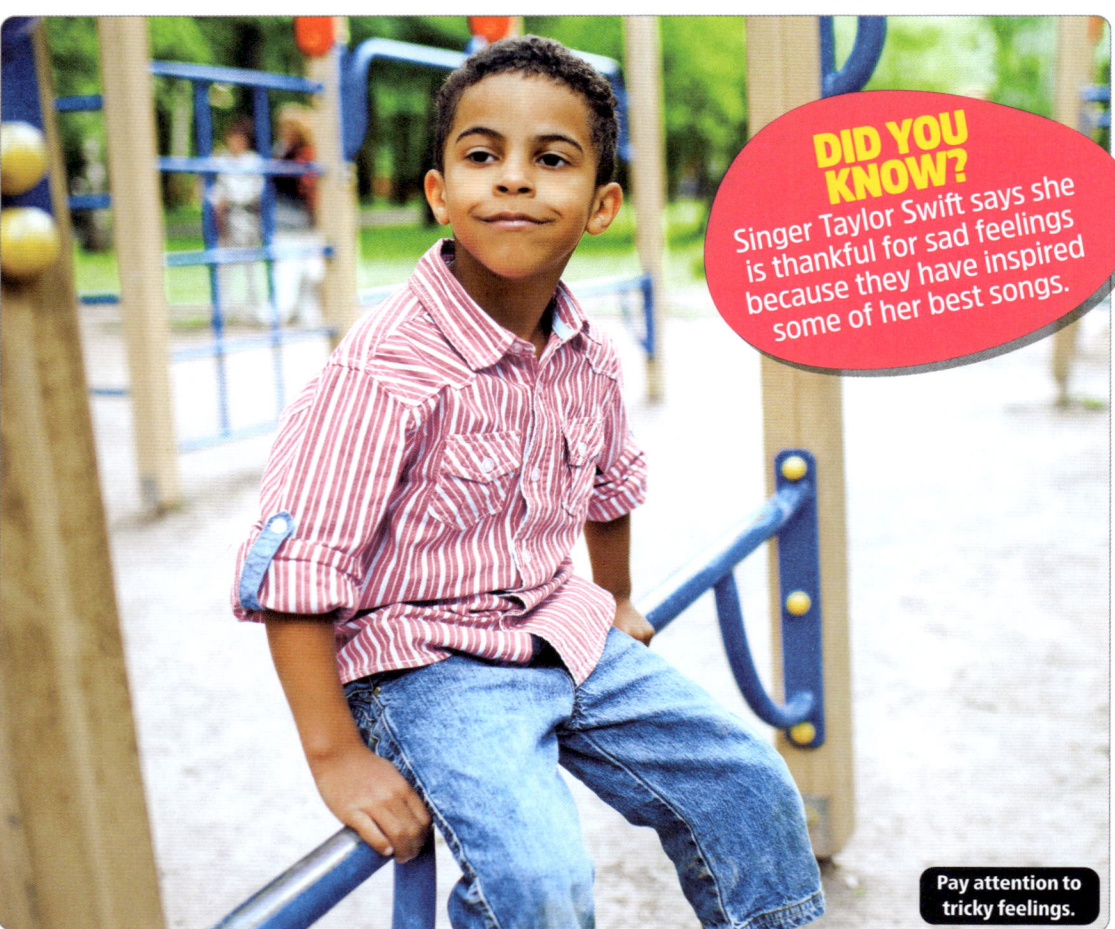

DID YOU KNOW? Singer Taylor Swift says she is thankful for sad feelings because they have inspired some of her best songs.

Pay attention to tricky feelings.

Imagine if you only felt so-called positive feelings, like excitement, joy, peace and safety. It might sound great but it's unrealistic. Being human means we experience all sorts of emotions, even ones that feel painful or uncomfortable (like anger, fear and sadness). Accepting these feelings is important and can improve your wellbeing.

Notice uncomfortable feelings
When you accept that difficult emotions are normal and temporary (they come and go, and will not last forever), you're often more able to cope with them. Psychologists are people who study the mind and human behaviour. They've found that people who allow themselves to feel a range of emotions, including painful ones, are often more at peace than people who try to avoid or push uncomfortable feelings away.

Does that mean all behaviour is ok?
If you allow yourself to feel anger, for example, that doesn't mean you can throw things around or behave unkindly. Anita Garai is a wellbeing teacher and author of *Being With Our Feelings*, a storybook collection. Garai says that if we allow ourselves to feel painful emotions, including anger, it's less likely these feelings will boil over and result in rash actions. "Uncomfortable feelings actually help to keep us well," she says. By listening to them, you can learn more about your needs and choose the best way to respond.

Sadness shows that you care.

How can I learn to accept uncomfortable feelings?
Garai suggests the first step is to simply notice and examine the uncomfortable feeling in your body. "Where in your body can you feel it? Is it still or moving? Can you describe the movement?" she says. It may be that the feeling reminds you of a colour, shape, sound or texture. By paying attention to the feeling in this way, it's less likely that you'll ignore it, explains Garai. Another tool is to read. Many people find it comforting and inspiring to read about characters (see top panel) who accept, manage and overcome tricky emotions by allowing these to simply exist.

Learn from others
Reading experts at Empathy Lab recommend these books.

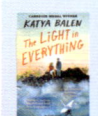

The Light in Everything by Katya Balen
Two children have to overcome anger, fear and sadness when they are thrown together in a newly blended family.

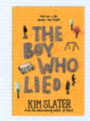

The Boy Who Lied by Kim Slater
Ed is ashamed of his family's poverty and lies to hide it. However, Ed discovers that telling the truth is an important way to build trust.

How difficult feelings can help you in life

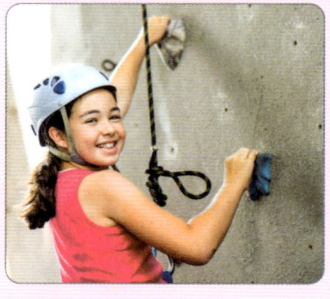

● **Fear**
Fear can prevent you from doing dangerous activities, keeping you safe. Sometimes, though, you'll need to take action despite your fear, which helps to build bravery.

● **Sadness**
Feeling sad is a signal that you care deeply about something. Expressing sadness, for example by crying, can make you feel lighter.

● **Anger**
Anger can be powerful. It can encourage you to stand up for yourself and to challenge unfairness when you see it.

● **Jealousy**
Feeling jealous can teach you about your own desires and inspire you to aim higher.

Accepting tricky feelings

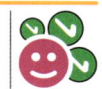

Feeling balloon
If we don't manage the build-up of emotions, just like a balloon, we will explode.

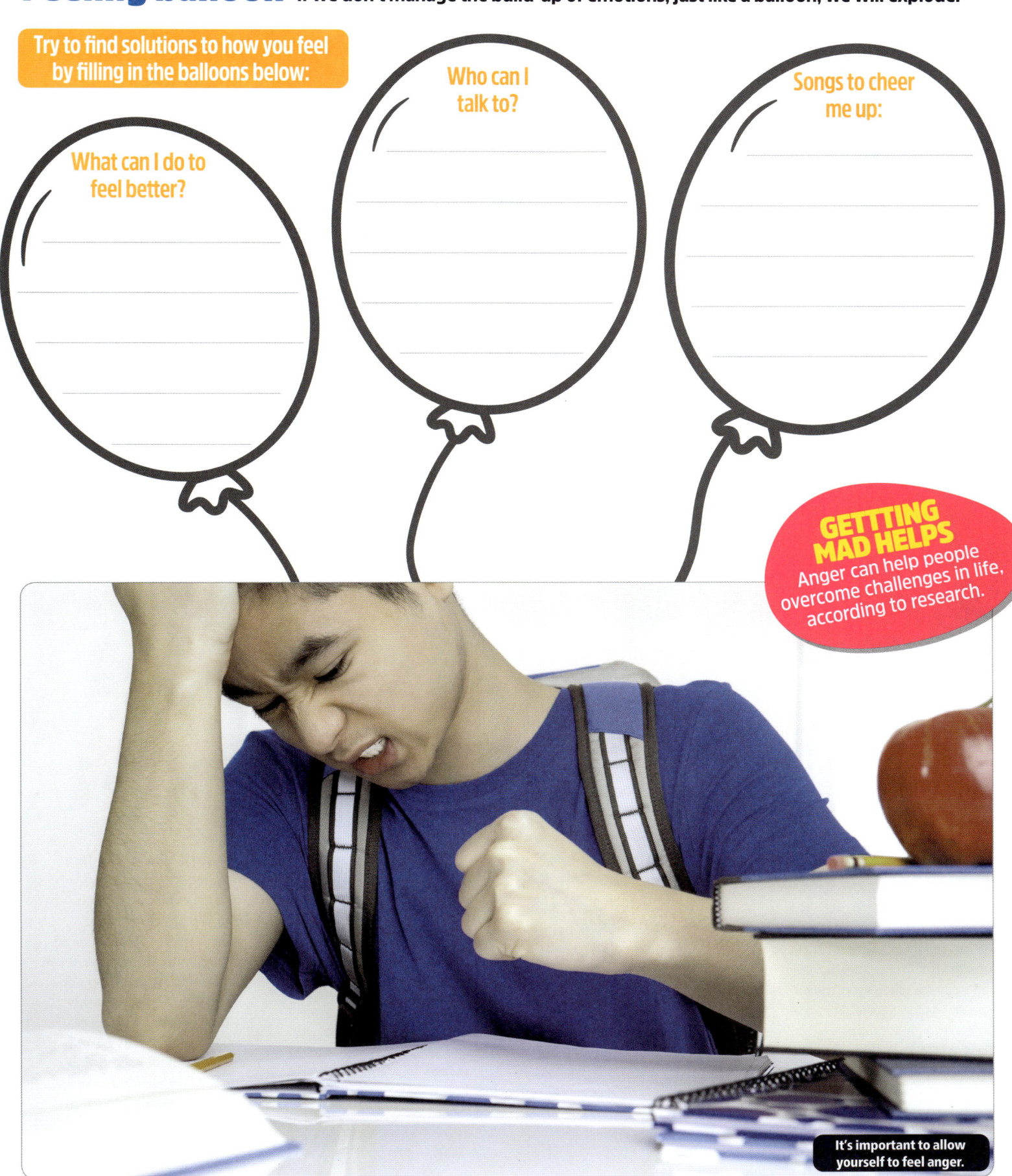

Try to find solutions to how you feel by filling in the balloons below:

What can I do to feel better?

Who can I talk to?

Songs to cheer me up:

GETTTING MAD HELPS
Anger can help people overcome challenges in life, according to research.

It's important to allow yourself to feel anger.

103

Emotional wellbeing

Dealing with drama

Learning to deal with difficult arguments can make you more confident.

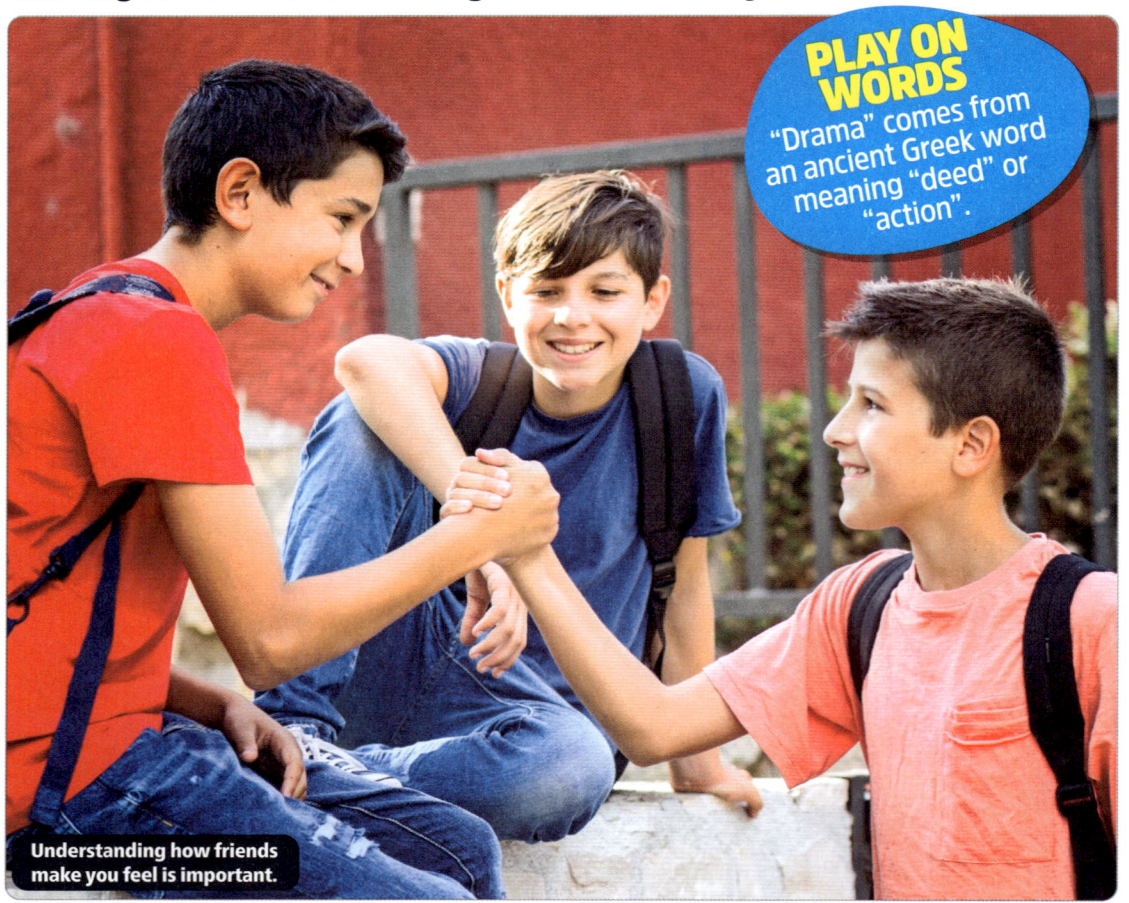

PLAY ON WORDS
"Drama" comes from an ancient Greek word meaning "deed" or "action".

Understanding how friends make you feel is important.

It's normal to argue with friends and siblings.

Have you ever fallen out with your friends? It's normal to have arguments and get on each other's nerves. Sometimes things can blow up into a drama and it can feel hard to put things right.

What is drama?
Drama means action and energy. It's exciting in a book or film but isn't always fun when it happens in real life. Falling out with someone and not knowing how to fix things can leave you feeling hurt, angry or upset. Psychologist (an expert on the brain and its functions) Dr Sara Carr explains that it's normal to fall out with friends sometimes. However, if an argument spirals out of control – especially if other people get involved – it can lead to drama. It can play out in school, online or in text messages. "Sometimes it's hard to know what to do if you become involved in drama," Carr says.

How does drama affect me?
Arguments can be upsetting, especially if you're sticking up for someone else or your words get misunderstood. Scientists say this causes your brain to release chemicals that make it hard to manage your emotions and can lead to you saying or doing things you might regret. This can also make you feel alone and lead to teasing or bullying. However, there are lots of ways to work through drama. Also, learning how to deal with friendship challenges helps you become more confident and handle arguments better in the future.

How to handle arguments
If you fall out with a friend, try talking about your feelings without involving other people, Carr says, as this could make things worse. Use statements starting with "I", like "I feel left out" instead of "You're leaving me out". Think about your values and what matters to you, such as kindness, to guide your actions. "How your friends make you feel is more important than how many friends you have," says Carr. If you feel an argument is too big to handle then sharing your concerns with a parent or teacher can help. Carr adds, "If talking is difficult, try writing something down instead."

Tips for making up after an argument
- Try to explain where you were coming from.
- If you feel you were wrong, say sorry.
- Make plans to do something fun and put the argument aside.
- Agree to disagree and try to move on, even if you can't find a solution for your argument.

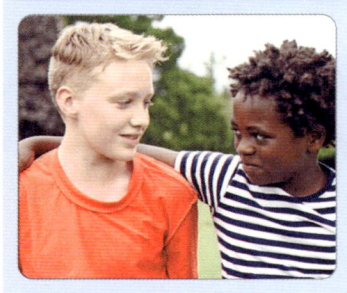

The difference between drama and bullying

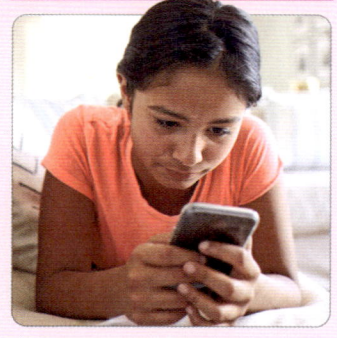

Bullying can be face-to-face or online (cyberbullying). It happens when a person or group of people make someone else feel frightened or bad about themselves. It can mean making fun of someone or repeatedly insulting them, telling lies about them or leaving them out of a group. Bullying is never acceptable and if it happens to you or someone else it's important to tell a trusted adult. You can find more advice about bullying at childline.org.uk

Dealing with drama

Write down what you want to say to someone in an argument in a letter. This will help you prepare to say it in person.

Emotional wellbeing

Learning to let go

Finding a way to forgive helps you leave bad feelings behind.

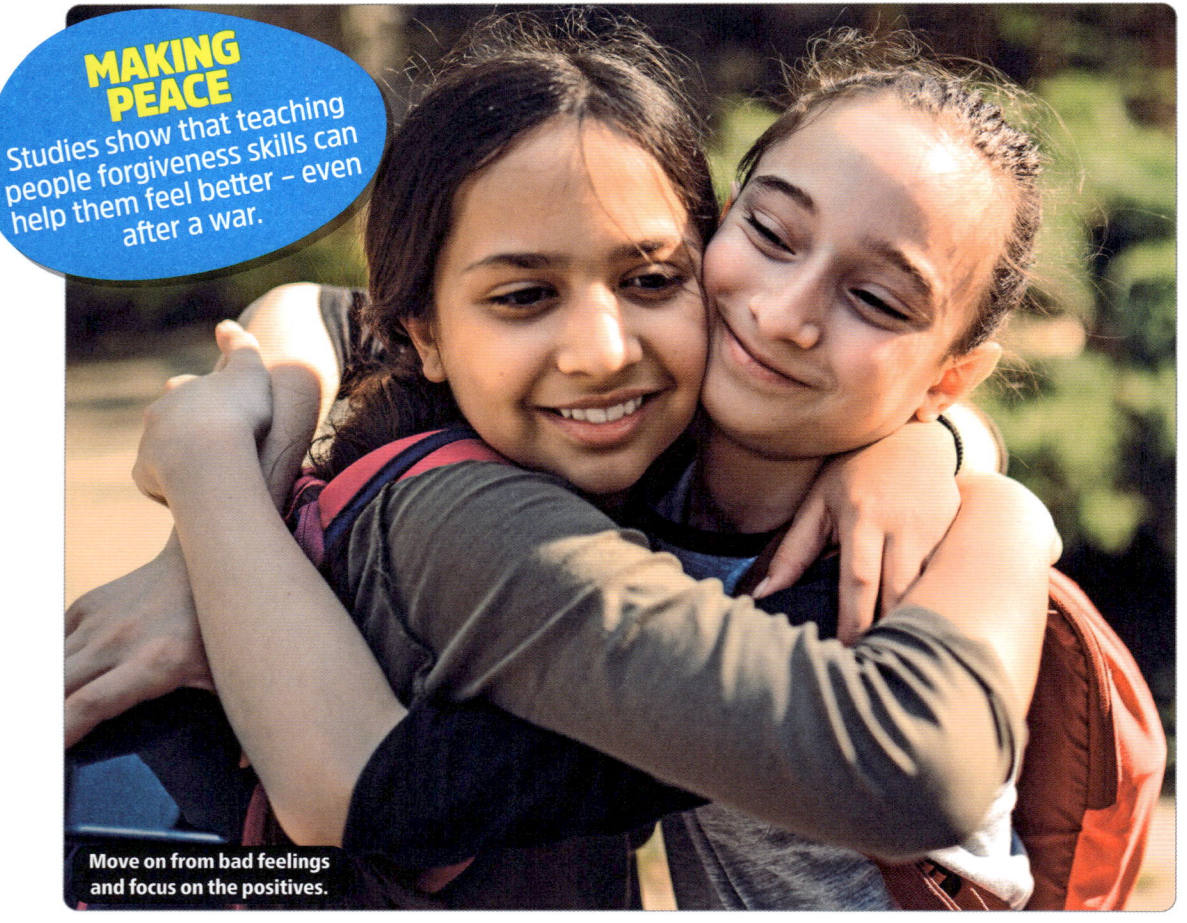

MAKING PEACE
Studies show that teaching people forgiveness skills can help them feel better – even after a war.

Move on from bad feelings and focus on the positives.

Everyone makes mistakes but if someone has hurt you it can be hard to forgive them and move on. Letting go of bad feelings helps you focus on your own happiness instead.

What is forgiveness?
Forgiveness means choosing to let go of anger towards someone who has hurt you. Say someone has behaved badly towards you, for example, by being mean or breaking your favourite game, forgiving them means deciding to let go of angry thoughts and move on. Author and forgiveness expert Fred Luskin says that forgiving someone doesn't mean forgetting or making excuses for what they've done. You don't need an apology to forgive and you don't have to make up with them. It involves finding the strength and courage to leave bad feelings behind and focus on yourself instead.

How does it benefit me?
Holding a grudge means holding on to hurt and anger, which isn't good for you. Scientists say letting go of these feelings makes you feel calmer, less stressed and can strengthen your immune system (how your body fights off illnesses). Learning to forgive involves trying to understand someone else's actions and putting yourself in their shoes. This is a good way to practise empathy (imagining someone else's feelings) and helps you to connect more closely with others.

Leave anger behind.

Can I learn to let go?
We can all learn to forgive but some find it easier than others. Luskin suggests focusing on how you feel. Instead of telling yourself something doesn't matter to you, try putting your feelings into words. You can do this by writing them down (see panel) or talking to someone that you trust. Don't expect your happiness to come from other people; find ways to make yourself happy instead, such as focusing on a new sport or hobby. Finally, don't waste time thinking about what someone else has said or done. "Put more energy into appreciating what you have," Luskin says. "Learn to look for the love, beauty and kindness around you."

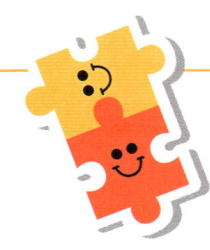

Tips for forgiving and being kinder to yourself

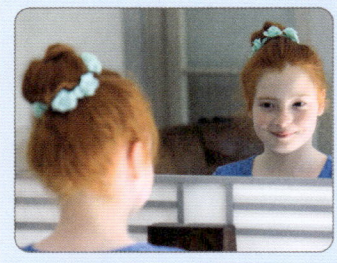

- Stand in front of a mirror and pretend you're forgiving someone else who's made the same mistake as you.
- Instead of feeling angry with yourself for failing a test or losing a sports match, focus on what you'll do differently next time.
- If you've made a mistake, write a list of good things that came out of it, however small they might be.
- Remember that forgiveness doesn't always happen straight away, it can take time and effort.

Focus on how you feel

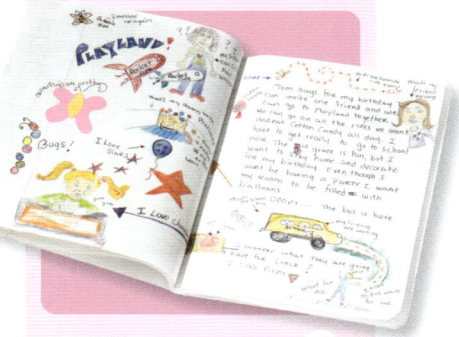

Journalling in a notebook is a great way to understand your thoughts and feelings. You can write words and draw pictures, patterns and squiggles. Try it every day, using pens, stickers and photos to share thoughts and feelings. You can even record poems or songs to express how you're feeling.

Learning to let go

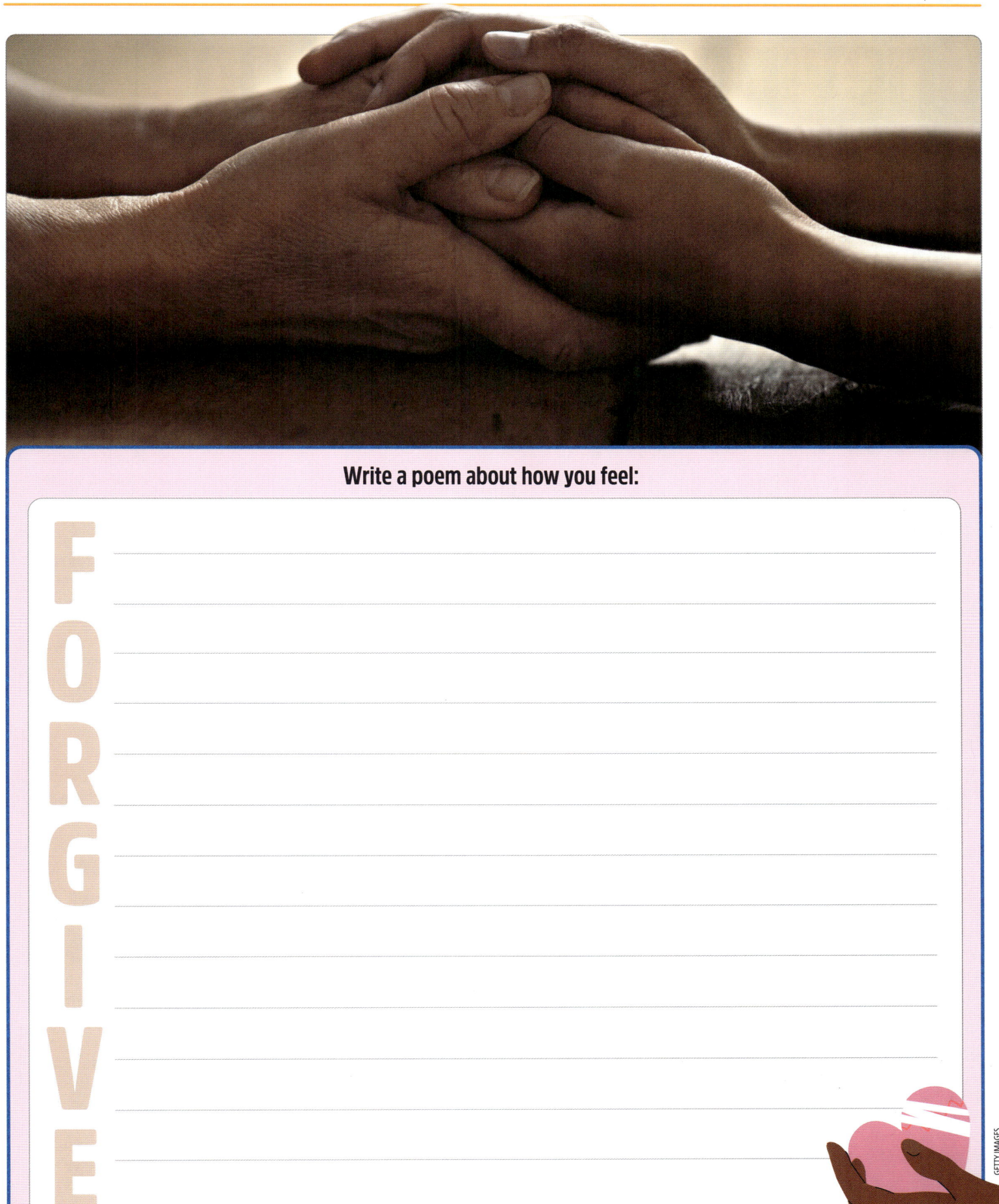

Write a poem about how you feel:

F
O
R
G
I
V
E

Emotional wellbeing

Grieving for a loved one

Talking about and celebrating your loved one's life helps.

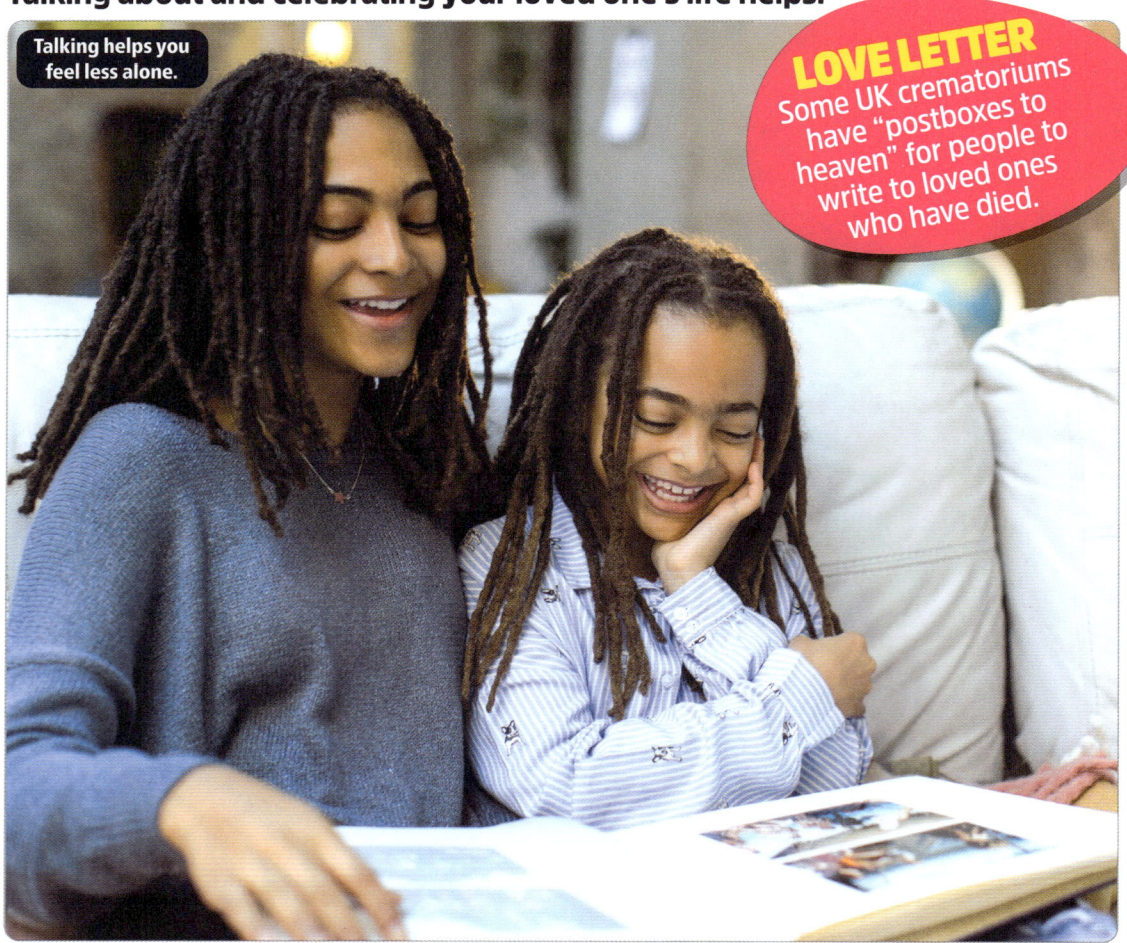

Talking helps you feel less alone.

LOVE LETTER
Some UK crematoriums have "postboxes to heaven" for people to write to loved ones who have died.

Make a memory box

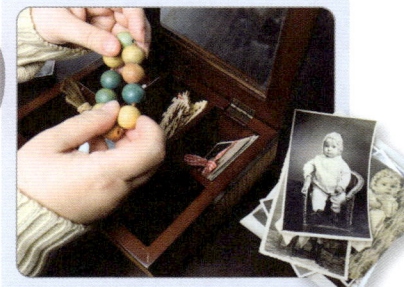

When a loved one has died it's important to remember and celebrate them. You can make a memory box that contains special items that remind you of them and what they mean to you. It could include photos, jewellery, letters, some of their things, mementos you've collected or tickets from places you visited together. You can use a shoe box and decorate it with paper, stickers or paint it in their favourite colour. Whenever you want to feel close to your loved one or talk about them, you can look inside your memory box.

When someone you care about dies, even when it's a person you didn't know, like somebody famous, you can feel lots of different and painful feelings. It can be difficult to deal with these feelings and know what to do with them. This is called grieving.

Coping with different feelings

When you grieve it's natural to feel sad, angry, anxious, guilty or numb. There may also be times when you feel happy or you laugh. There isn't one way you should feel when somebody dies; whatever you're feeling is ok.

Grief coach Rebecca-Monique says when a person you care about dies your relationship with them doesn't disappear, it just changes. "Feelings want your attention. It helps to notice them, name them and talk about them. This way they don't stay bottled up. Talking about your loved one who has died can help other people learn about how special they were to you, and makes you feel less alone in grief. Talking about them is also a way of honouring their life – the fact they existed and still do, in your heart."

Listening can help a grieving friend.

Celebrate occasions without them

Special dates like birthdays, festivals and family gatherings can feel tricky when your loved one is no longer there. Rebecca-Monique says that it's normal to feel guilty if you celebrate and try your best to carry on with life, and that this doesn't make you a bad person. "You can make sure the memory of your loved one is included in the celebration by creating traditions and rituals like wearing their favourite colour or observing a minute's silence. You may want to avoid occasions because the thought of your loved one not physically being with you is still too painful. It's fine to sit it out if it feels too much."

Talk to a grieving friend

When a friend is grieving you may struggle to know what to say. Pretending nothing has happened doesn't help your friend. Asking if they'd like to talk about how they feel shows you care. If they get upset that's ok, it's natural to be emotional. You don't have to fix anything or make them feel better, just listening and being there will mean a lot to your friend.

"I'd tell other young people to talk about it"

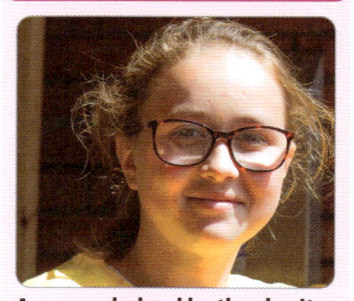

Amy was helped by the charity Child Bereavement UK after her dad died when she was 11. She says, "I'd tell other young people in the same situation as me to talk about it. It seems really hard to start off with, but, when you talk to other people about it, you might feel upset, but they'll know the reason why and they'll comfort you."
Amy, aged 14

108

Grieving for a loved one

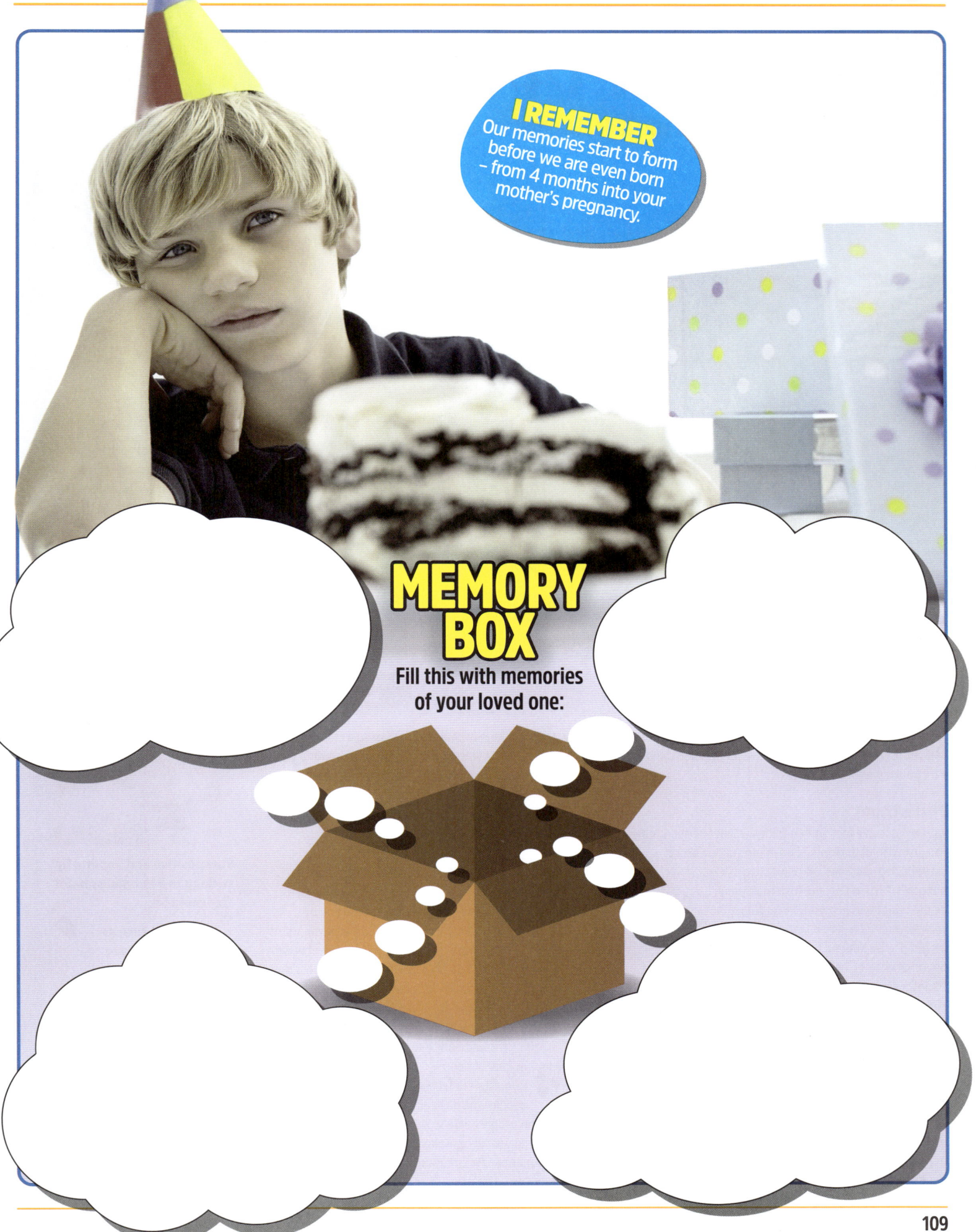

I REMEMBER
Our memories start to form before we are even born – from 4 months into your mother's pregnancy.

MEMORY BOX
Fill this with memories of your loved one:

Emotional wellbeing

The power of hope

Keeping a sense of hope helps you to feel calm and happy.

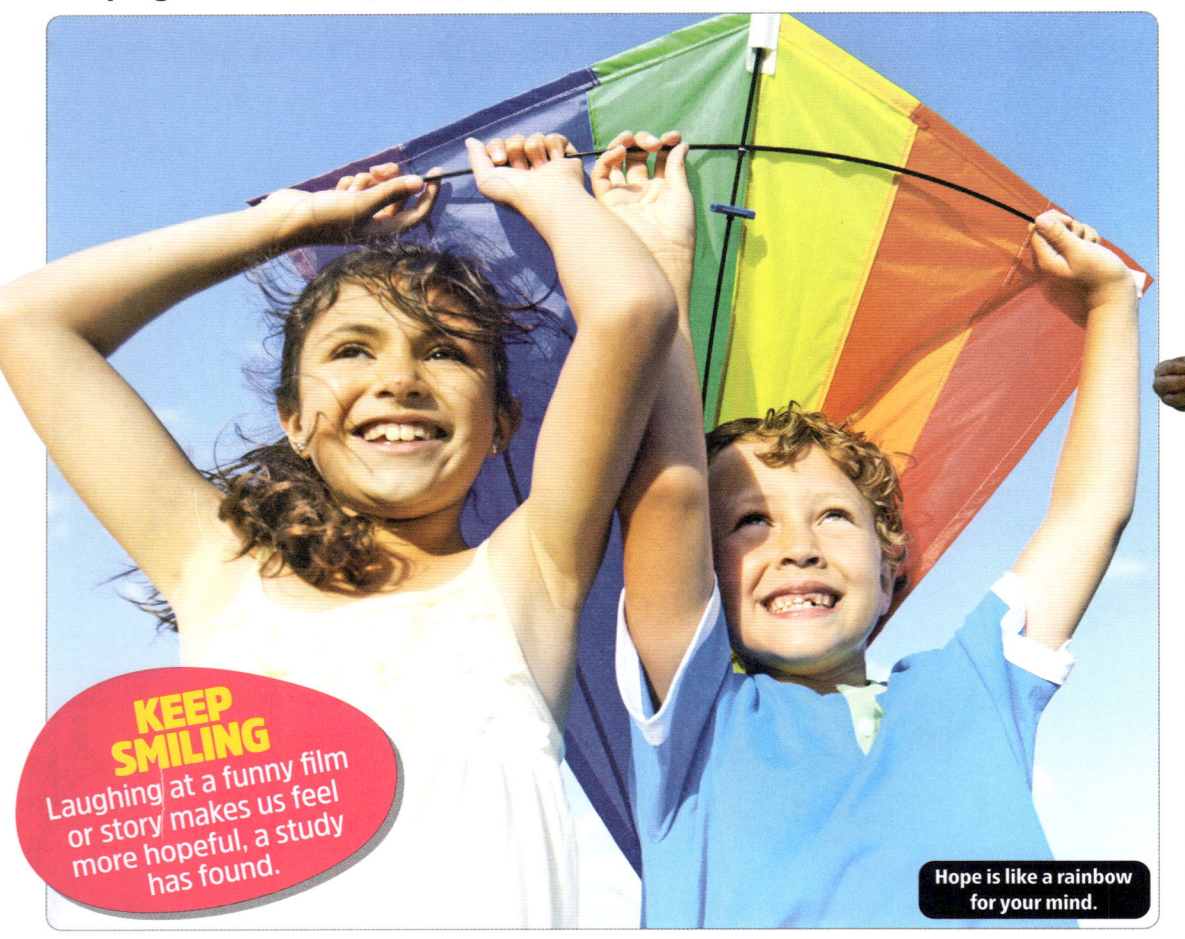

KEEP SMILING
Laughing at a funny film or story makes us feel more hopeful, a study has found.

Hope is like a rainbow for your mind.

Being hopeful is a powerful feeling. This is because hope gives us the strength to be positive, even when things don't go our way.

What is hope?
Hope is a positive feeling that things will get better. It's more than just wishful thinking; hope means taking action and believing you have the power to achieve your goals. "When I'm hopeful it makes me see the brightness in myself," says *The Week Junior* reader Jonah, aged eight, "It's good to be hopeful because it gives you a chance to be happy about things." Charles Snyder, a psychologist (an expert in how we think) studied hopeful thinking and said it has three main parts: having a goal, thinking up different ways to achieve it and believing in yourself even when things go wrong.

How is hope good for me?
Snyder called hope a "rainbow of the mind," because it "lifts our spirits and makes us think of what is possible". Being hopeful about something, like trying out a new sport or hobby, takes courage because you're taking a step into the unknown. This helps you work out what's important to you, as well as making you more confident and resilient (able to overcome challenges). Studies show that being hopeful also helps you learn better at school, build strong friendships and feel less stressed.

Jonah says hope can help you to be happy.

How can I be more hopeful?
Hope is a skill you can learn. Hope expert David Feldman suggests starting by working towards a goal that's important to you, then thinking up different ways to achieve it. So if you hope to be a chef one day, for example, aim to learn one new recipe a week. Staying focused on your goal takes energy, so Feldman recommends eating healthily and getting plenty of sleep.
If you start to feel hopeless, get inspired by people who have already succeeded or tell someone who supports you so they can give you a boost. Finally, tap into your imagination and picture yourself achieving your goal. Picturing success in the future is hope in action.

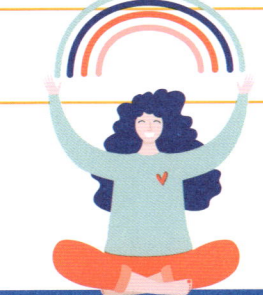

Create a hope cloud

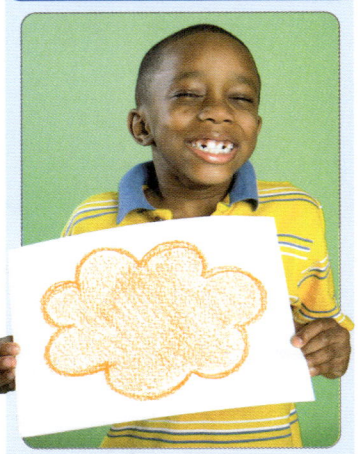

Think about something you hope for and write it in a cloud shape. Then write at least one thing you can do to get closer to your dream and someone you could ask for help. Keep the cloud where you can see it to remind you to stay hopeful in reaching your dream.

Happiness habits

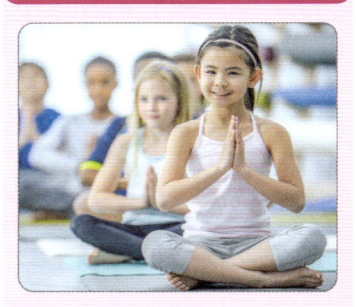

Stay positive and hopeful by sticking to a happiness habit. This could be:

- **Exercising, such as practising yoga or organising a football match with friends.**
- **Playing or listening to music.**
- **Volunteering to help others – for example, helping a neighbour with their garden.**
- **Spending time in nature by going for a walk or bike ride.**

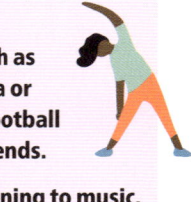

The power of hope

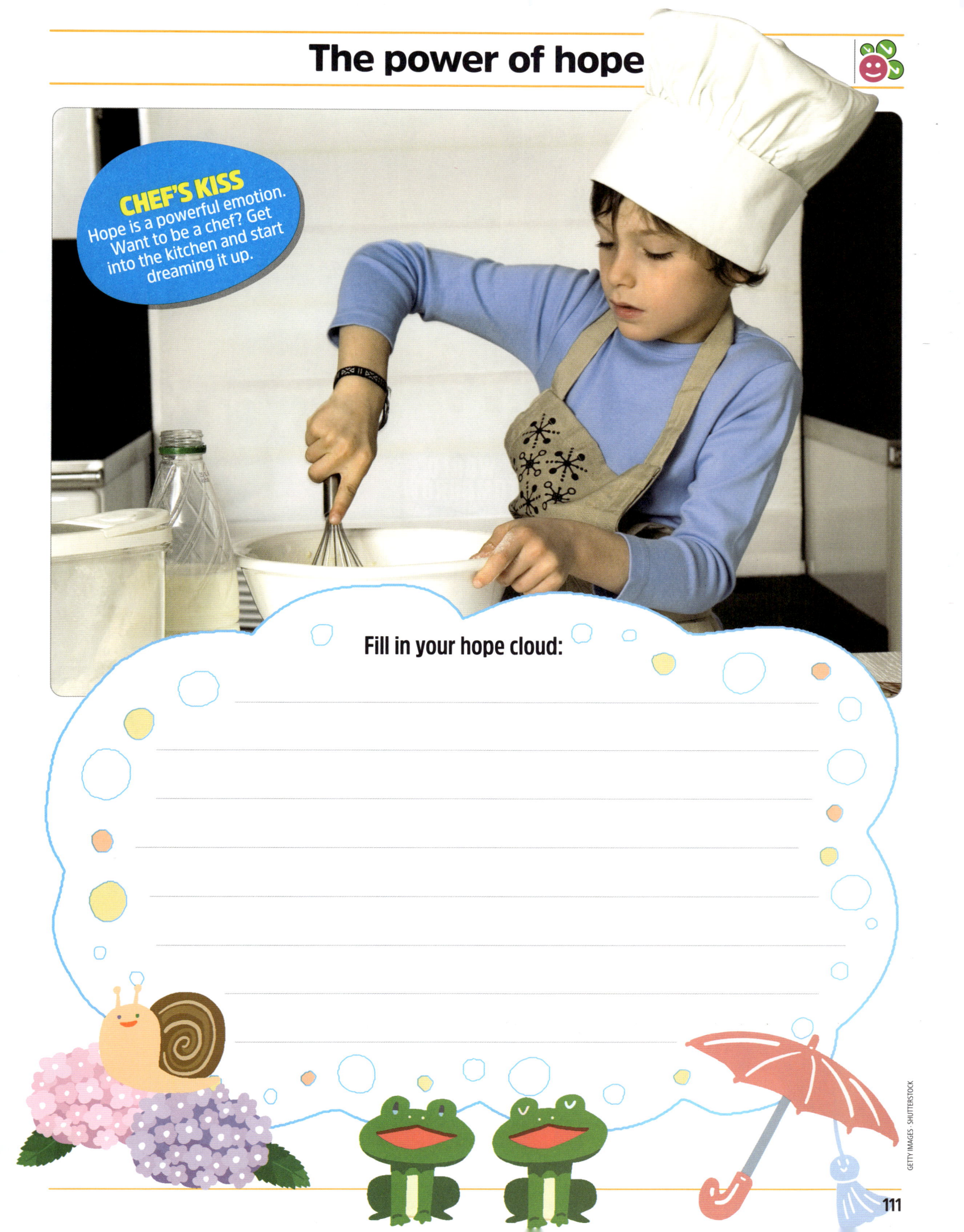

CHEF'S KISS
Hope is a powerful emotion. Want to be a chef? Get into the kitchen and start dreaming it up.

Fill in your hope cloud:

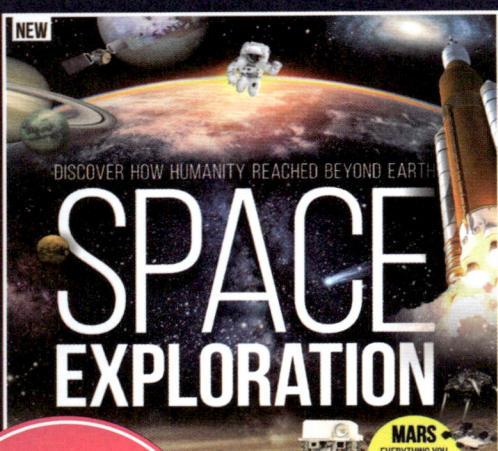

Find out everything you've ever wanted to know about outer space

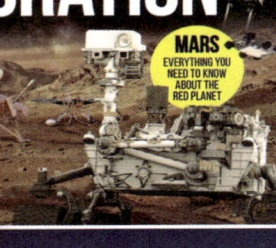

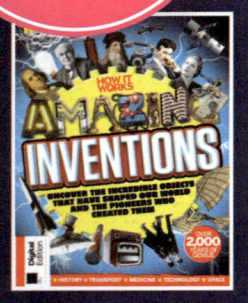

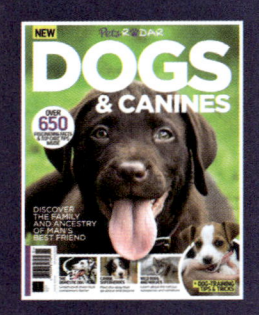

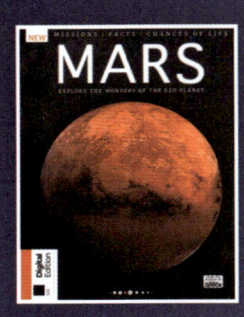

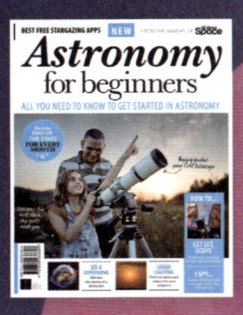

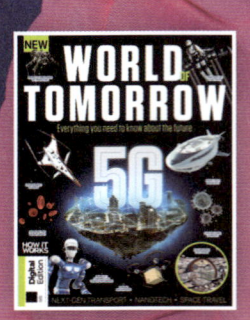

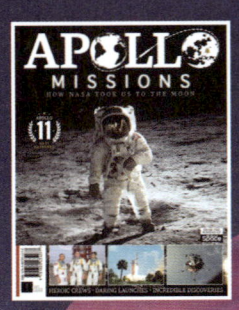

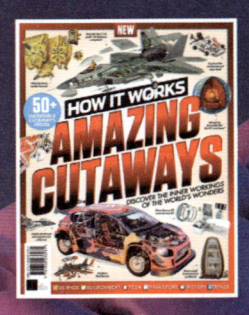

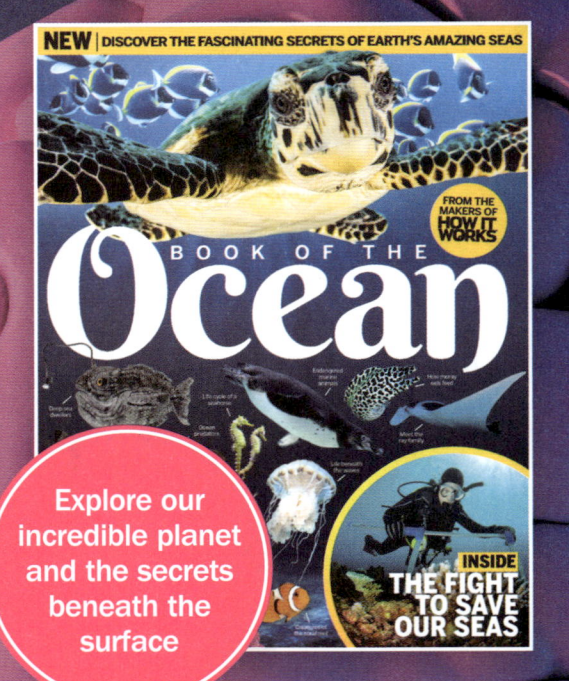

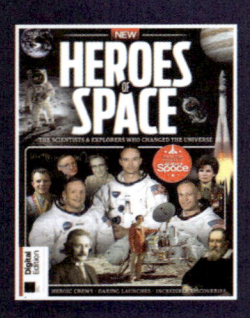

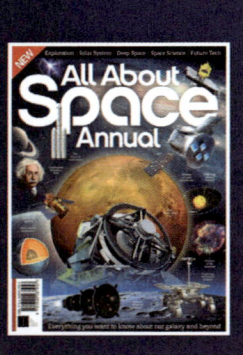

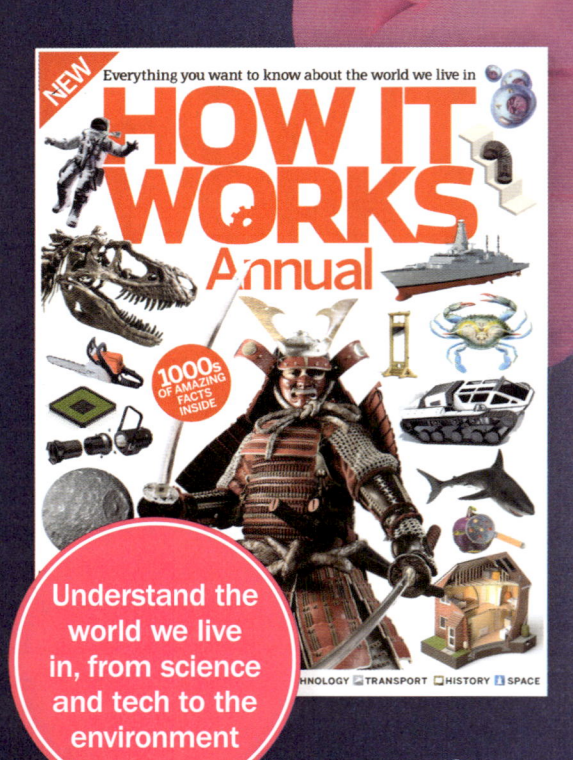

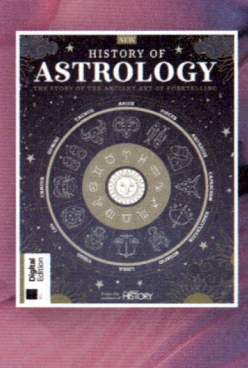

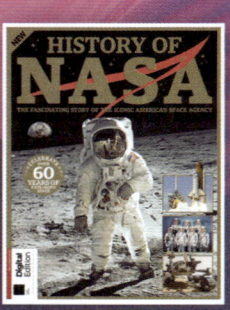

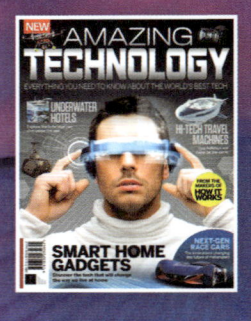

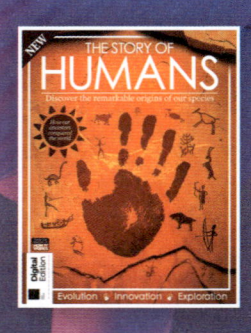

Explore our incredible planet and the secrets beneath the surface

Understand the world we live in, from science and tech to the environment

✓ Get great savings when you buy direct from us

✓ 1000s of great titles, many not available anywhere else

✓ World-wide delivery and super-safe ordering

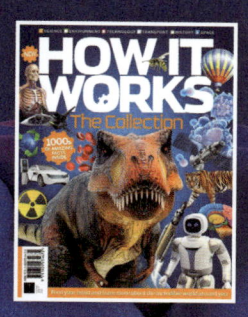

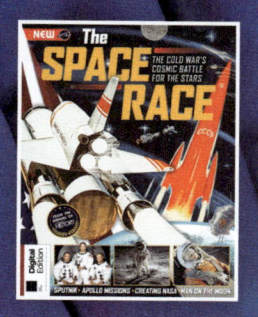

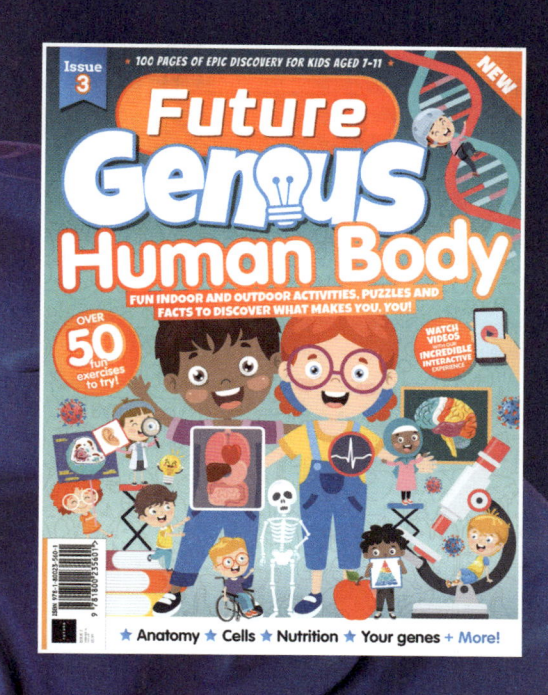

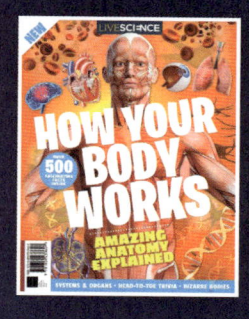

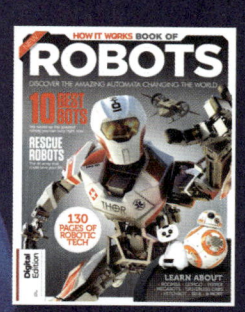

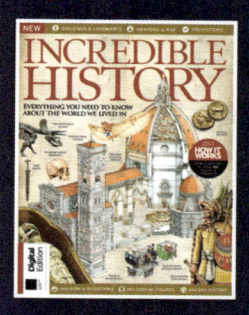

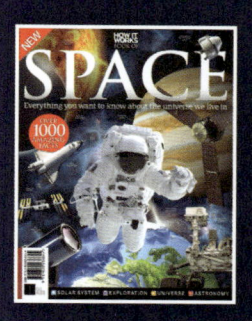

FEED YOUR MIND WITH OUR BOOKAZINES

Explore the secrets of the universe, from the days of the dinosaurs to the miracles of modern science!

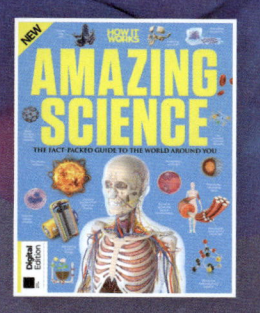

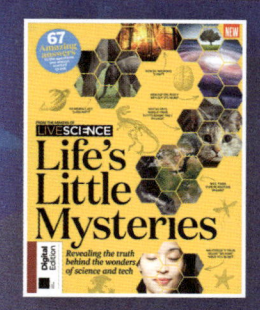

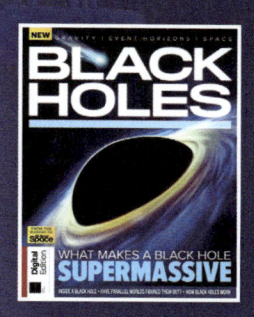

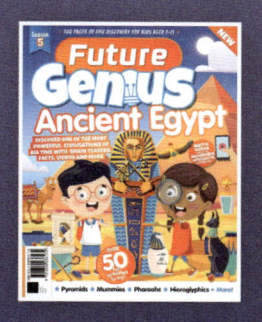

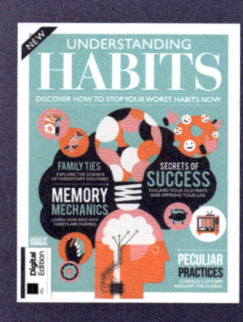

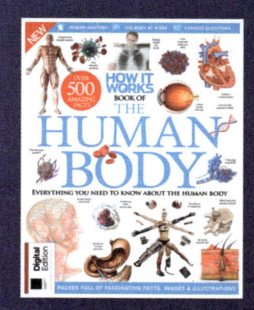

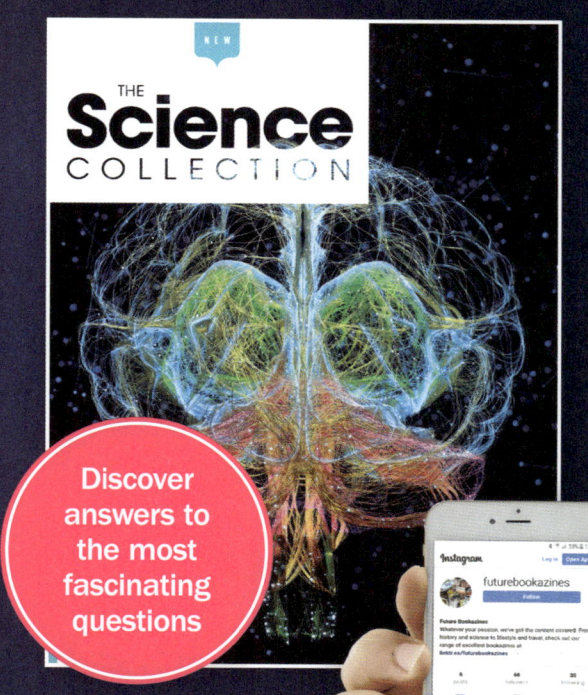

Discover answers to the most fascinating questions

Follow us on Instagram 📷 @futurebookazines

www.magazinesdirect.com
Magazines, back issues & bookazines.

FUTURE

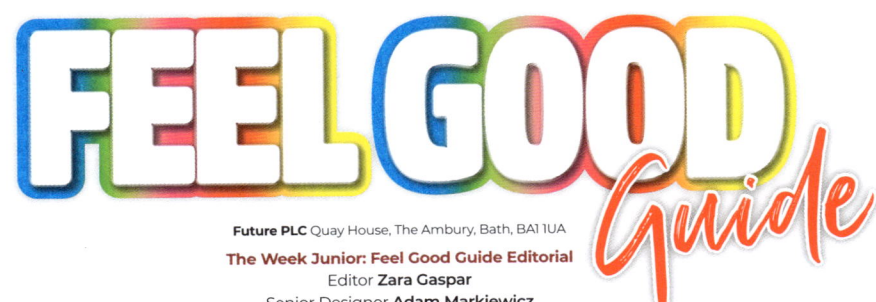

FEEL GOOD Guide

Future PLC Quay House, The Ambury, Bath, BA1 1UA

The Week Junior: Feel Good Guide Editorial
Editor **Zara Gaspar**
Senior Designer **Adam Markiewicz**
Head of Art & Design **Greg Whitaker**
Editorial Director **Jon White**
Managing Director **Grainne McKenna**

The Week Junior Editorial
Editor **Dan Green**
Designers **Heather Reeves, Philip Allardice**
Editorial Director **Anna Bassi**
Group Art Director **Dave Kelsall**

Contributors
Lucy Mason

Cover images
Getty, Alamy, Shutterstock

Photography
All copyrights and trademarks are recognised and respected

Advertising
Media packs are available on request
Commercial Director **Clare Dove**

International
Head of Print Licensing **Rachel Shaw**
licensing@futurenet.com
www.futurecontenthub.com

Circulation
Head of Newstrade **Tim Mathers**

Production
Head of Production **Mark Constance**
Production Project Manager **Matthew Eglinton**
Advertising Production Manager **Joanne Crosby**
Digital Editions Controller **Jason Hudson**
Production Managers **Keely Miller, Nola Cokely, Vivienne Calvert, Fran Twentyman**

Printed in the UK

Distributed by Marketforce – www.marketforce.co.uk
For enquiries, please email: mfcommunications@futurenet.com

Feel Good Guide First Edition (WJB6310)
© 2024 Future Publishing Limited

We are committed to only using magazine paper which is derived from responsibly managed, certified forestry and chlorine-free manufacture. The paper in this bookazine was sourced and produced from sustainable managed forests, conforming to strict environmental and socioeconomic standards.

All contents © 2024 Future Publishing Limited or published under licence. All rights reserved. No part of this magazine may be used, stored, transmitted or reproduced in any way without the prior written permission of the publisher. Future Publishing Limited (company number 2008885) is registered in England and Wales. Registered office: Quay House, The Ambury, Bath BA1 1UA. All information contained in this publication is for information only and is, as far as we are aware, correct at the time of going to press. Future cannot accept any responsibility for errors or inaccuracies in such information. You are advised to contact manufacturers and retailers directly with regard to the price of products/services referred to in this publication. Apps and websites mentioned in this publication are not under our control. We are not responsible for their contents or any other changes or updates to them. This magazine is fully independent and not affiliated in any way with the companies mentioned herein.

FUTURE Connectors. Creators. Experience Makers.

Future plc is a public company quoted on the London Stock Exchange (symbol: FUTR)
www.futureplc.com

Chief Executive Officer **Jon Steinberg**
Non-Executive Chairman **Richard Huntingford**
Chief Financial and Strategy Officer **Penny Ladkin-Brand**

Tel +44 (0)1225 442 244

Part of the
THE WEEK Junior Making sense of the world
bookazine series

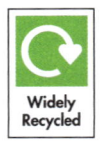

Widely Recycled | ipso For press freedom with responsibility